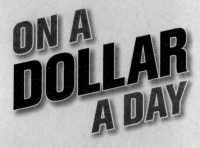

ON A DOLLAR A DAY

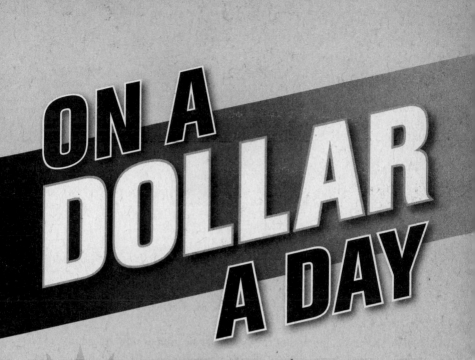

One Couple's Unlikely Adventures in Eating in America

CHRISTOPHER GREENSLATE
KERRI LEONARD

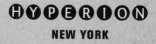

HYPERION

NEW YORK

Copyright © 2010 Christopher Greenslate and Kerri Leonard

Library of Congress Cataloging-in-Publication Data has been applied for.

ISBN 978-1-4013-1018-9

Hyperion books are available for special promotions, premiums, or
corporate training. For details contact the HarperCollins Special Markets
Department in the New York office at 212-207-7528, fax 212-207-7222, or
e-mail spsales@harpercollins.com.

Design by Renato Stanisic

FIRST EDITION

10 9 8 7 6 5 4 3 2 1

To our parents, for feeding us

Contents

Part III—Striving to Eat Healthfully

PART I
THE ONE DOLLAR DIET PROJECT

Priced Out

As we walked out of the grocery store, I told Christopher, "You need to stop doing that."

"Doing what?" he asked.

"Telling people about the dollar-a-day thing. It's weird. And we're weird enough already."

"Okay, but I don't think it's that big of a deal."

I disagreed. It *was* a big deal, and it was weird. I was up for the challenge, but I didn't think the whole world needed to know about our experiment. Little did I know what was in store.

The idea to reduce the cost of our diet to a dollar each per day had been simmering since May, when Christopher and I had gone grocery shopping and I was feeling financially stretched. The bounty of colorful, fresh organic produce and the southern California sunlight coming through the large windows of Jimbo's, our local natural foods store, was not enough to massage away my economic stress. The number at the bottom of the register tape seemed higher than usual; several people had been over to our house for dinner during the past few weeks, and I always cook something special for guests. We want people to enjoy memorable food when they eat with us, but it gets expensive.

On top of that, we were approaching the end of the school year. As public high school teachers, we only get paychecks eleven months out of the year. We bought a house the previous summer, and I felt even more apprehensive about making the mortgage than I had the year before. Saving throughout the year is a challenge, and our teachers' salaries don't leave us much room to be frivolous with our funds. Car payments, mortgage payments, and credit card payments all marched through my mind as I tallied up our food bill. Christopher doesn't worry about the summer like I do. He manages to keep his finances in order, but I have the burden of credit card debt and school loans weighing upon me. I felt as if I would never get out from under it.

We arrived home from the store on that May afternoon and I dropped the brimming canvas shopping bags onto the kitchen counter. While we put away the groceries, I complained about the cost of our shopping trip and told Christopher that we needed to find a way to spend less on food. My proposed solutions ran along the lines of more reasonable grocery lists and better planning. I should have known that Christopher would have something to add. He typically responds in a way that both enlightens and annoys me. That was when he volunteered the information that a large portion of the world eats on a dollar a day or less.

"Why don't we try it?" he asked.

I rolled my eyes. Pretty soon he would be talking about Bangladesh or some other developing nation that we should learn from. All I wanted was to crawl out from under the weight of my economic woes, not hear about people halfway around the world. Yet when Christopher goes on about things like this, there are times when he convinces me to look at what we have differently. At times it was exhausting, but sometimes we changed what we were doing. This was one of those moments when I ended up agreeing. We would try it; we would eat on a dollar each a day.

I never expected that, when I met the man of my dreams, my eating habits would be transformed. Christopher and I had met four years before in our teaching credential program. I had moved to San

Diego only a few months earlier and didn't know many people. During our first class, one of our teachers explained that we'd spend a great deal of time together. He added that over the years several couples had resulted from the program. I looked around the room and could not picture these people dating each other. I never would have guessed that I would be the first.

However, Christopher intrigued me from the start. As we toured the campus, I noticed the cute guy with the dark hair and black-rimmed glasses. The "Go Vegan" button on his messenger bag further compelled me to pay attention. I had attempted vegetarianism a few times during my college years, but I had one roommate whom we jokingly referred to as the "Beef Princess," and another who felt that the only vegetables worth eating were corn and potatoes, so my attempts were doomed. However, a year or two earlier I had eliminated all red meat from my diet and ate only chicken and, on rare occasions, fish. This vegan boy in my class made me feel inspired to try again, and this time I succeeded. Christopher always made sure that our assignments were tied in to what was going on in the world, and it was obvious that he was on a mission to make a difference. We began flirting within a week or two, and I was smitten. When I talked to my roommates, I referred to him as "my vegan boyfriend," but I never imagined that he was interested in me.

One evening in October, about six weeks into our program, I turned on my computer to find an e-mail from a classmate. She informed me that Christopher would not stop talking about me, and that I should give him a chance. She added the selling point that he could cook. Within a week, we were inseparable. In January, he came with me to northern California to meet my family, and by the time we went home I was vegan. I thought it would be frustrating to try to figure out what to eat when I was choosing to avoid not only meat but all dairy and eggs as well, but the transition wasn't hard.

Christopher had been vegan for almost seven years. There is a myth that eating vegan is difficult. If students find out I am vegan, they ask, "What do you eat?" One student even made the comment, "You must not like food." Most people ask the standard questions:

Where do you get your protein? Are you healthy? Don't you ever just want to quit and eat a hamburger? And they make standard assumptions: Vegan food tastes bad, you must crave cheese, and there is no way you can get all of your nutrients. The reality is that making a switch to a plant-based diet is not as difficult as one may think. In hindsight, compared to the dollar-a-day diet, it was one of the easiest changes I have made.

Despite the fact that I agreed to the dollar plan, I was reluctant. During the school year, Christopher makes our lunches every day, and on the weekends he often whips up some French toast or chocolate chip pancakes. I am usually in charge of planning the shopping lists and preparing dinner, and I worried that this new endeavor would add too much work to our routine. I wasn't sure I was ready for the commitment, and I didn't want to simply trade economic uneasiness for culinary difficulties.

In addition, we both had a lot going on that summer. Christopher would be gone for three weeks on a journalism fellowship and a residency to complete his master's degree. I would be home teaching summer school for the first three weeks. After that, we were both headed for my family's annual vacation. Then the week before we had to report back to work was Christopher's birthday, and we had planned a camping trip at Yellowstone National Park. We tossed around different times to start our "dollar diet," but it seemed like summer was out of the question. So we decided to start in September.

Summer came, and we talked a lot about the plan to eat for less. I told my parents and my closest friends, but Christopher told everyone. That's just how he is. When he gets the chance, he will talk to anyone willing to listen to his ideas. Each time "the experiment" came up, I shrank into my shoes, trying to find a way to end the conversation or run interference and take it in a different direction. He wanted to involve everyone in the discourse; I did not want our quirkiness to be the focus. But what we found was that the conversation always moved away from what *we* were doing and into discussions on poverty, food prices, grocery shopping, and farming:

everything and anything related to food. People told us about tough times when they struggled with food issues of their own. This was what got Christopher motivated; he reads everything he can get his hands on and absorbs it into his thinking. I admit that it was fascinating to hear what other people had to say. I even learned about the problems that my own parents had faced when they were young.

As an English major, I hadn't planned on food becoming the focus of my life. Ask me about Dostoevsky and we're in business, but bring up food stamp allocation, third-world debt, or the modern global food system, and I do my best just to tread water. But the conversations about food and economics were interesting. As for our project, we had no concrete plans or expertise that would help us to actually carry it out. We only knew that it would involve guesswork and trial and error. We planned to purchase foods in bulk, but we weren't sure what specific items or what meals would come from it. Our summer left little time to actually investigate.

When I went home to visit my best friend, Nicole, she and I laughed with my parents about what we would eat and how it would work. We joked about having a monochromatic diet—white foods, lots of flour, potatoes, and rice. Although they laughed, I could tell that my parents were concerned. They were worried that we would get sick or lose too much weight. I wasn't as bothered by those issues as I was with the thought of being hungry. I hate the feeling of my stomach growling and churning. If I skip a meal, I get grouchy and short-tempered. I like to experiment with recipes, try new foods. In short, I like to cook and I like to eat. We have at least twenty cookbooks, and I love digging through them to find different treats. During the school year, we get caught up in a rotation of basic meals, but in the summer I try to break out of the pattern and make at least one new meal each week. We move our quick favorites to our workweek lineup, saving the time-consuming meals for special occasions.

As we sat around my parents' kitchen table, in the home where I spent most of my childhood, I realized that eating out would soon be impossible. We eat most of our meals at home, but we do frequent a few local restaurants. Ask anyone from Southern California and they're bound to have their own favorite taco shop. Rico's is ours, a favorite of Christopher's since his high school days. Christopher introduced me to this burrito haven located at the east end of our sleepy beach town when we first started dating, and it would be accurate to say that we have a bit of a love affair with Rico's. In fact, this special place was where I learned that a side of French fries and a burrito complement each other in ways that I still do not understand. When Christopher and I met, it quickly became our weekly date after our Monday night class. Once we started teaching, it became the "it's Friday and we don't want to cook" spot. However, with only a dollar each to spend, Rico's was out.

Cookbook browsing and fine dining would have to be put on hold for a month. We would need to change the way we looked at food. No longer would we be able to eat based on taste; our guts would be governed by our pocketbooks. This was not necessarily a bad thing, as we both have a tendency to overeat. We often eat until we are full, uncomfortably so. When I cook, I make a lot of food, and I don't serve small portions. I have difficulty making salads because while lettuce and tomatoes are great together, they seem to taste better when you add kidney and garbanzo beans, avocado, carrots, cucumber, bell peppers, sprouts, and any other vegetable that we might have. After a while, my salads become large enough to feed six or seven people. I do the same thing when preparing meals. At least now we would be forced to eat reasonably sized servings.

I had spent quite a bit of time that summer considering what we would have to do without, but it was not until we returned home from our camping trip near the end of August that we started figuring out what we would have to work with. Christopher had ordered the book *Eat Well on a Dollar a Day* by Bill and Ruth Kaysing for—no kidding—one dollar. It had arrived while we were camping. It was older than we were and did not look like most cookbooks or healthy living guides, but it reaffirmed what we planned to do. The book outlined some key strategies for making every penny count: buy in bulk, shop around, eat smaller portions, and forage. In addition to taking this crash course in frugal living, we also had scheduled our annual health checkups. We told our doctor about the plan; he seemed unfazed. He mentioned that we would probably lose some weight, but if we were taking multivitamins, then it should not be harmful. At that point we planned to continue taking vitamins, so we felt reassured.

The first hint I had of the challenges in store for us came when we returned from Yellowstone to a virtually empty kitchen cupboard. On several occasions when we returned home, I mentioned that we needed to get groceries, but every time Christopher shot down my suggestion. One evening around dinnertime we had no food in the house, or so I thought. I hunted around in the cabinets trying to figure out what to eat. I could see the sun setting over the backyard fence and our dogs, Viola and Horatio, wrestling in the dirt. I again attempted to convince Christopher to run to the store, a five-minute jaunt in the car, but Christopher said that he wanted us to finish off the food we had left before we started our project. That was easy for him to say; he didn't have to make a meal from what seemed to be nothing. Despite his resistance to going shopping, he offered no solutions to our problem. When I said I would go to the store alone, he argued that there was plenty in the house if I just changed the way I looked at what we had.

I began slamming cupboard doors, but Christopher was unmoved. I complained that we had peanut butter, but no jelly, and no bread. We had one can of beans and a little bit of lettuce, but no tortillas or any other taco fixings. We had one can of split pea soup, which Christopher loves, but I don't. I felt that any rational person would have agreed that a trip to the store was in order, but Christopher is not a normal person.

"Millions of people make their own tortillas every day. We're probably smart enough to figure it out," he said.

Sometimes I hate it when he's right, but we looked up tortilla recipes online and, sure enough, within thirty minutes we were cooking. When I realized that burritos would be possible during our project, I knew I would survive.

It was about this time that we agreed upon our rules for the project. We didn't want so many that we couldn't eat anything, but we wanted guidelines, so we came up with five that we could live with:

1. **All food consumed each day had to total not more than one dollar for each of us.**
2. **We could not accept free food or "donated" food unless it was available for everyone in our area (e.g., foraging, samples from stores, Dumpster diving).**
3. **Any vegetables we planted in our garden, we had to pay for (i.e., seeds or potted plants).**
4. **We would do our best to cook a variety of meals; we would only eat ramen noodles if there was no other way to stay under one dollar. (We had six packages of ramen, and would buy no more.)**
5. **If we decided to have guests over for dinner, they had to eat from our share, meaning they didn't get their own dollar's worth of food.**

The donated food rule was a necessity. My family lives ten hours away, but Christopher's family lives close by. Both his mom and sister suggested that it would not be cheating if someone *happened* to leave bags of food or plates of cookies outside our front door. They argued that we didn't pay for it, so we didn't have to figure it into our costs. However, we thought that would be cheating. If we allowed people to leave us food or cook for us, we could probably get ourselves fed most evenings by friends or family. People who are truly poor wouldn't have that resource. We eventually convinced them that even if they left the food, it would rot on our doorstep.

The rule that we would pay for vegetables that we planted ended up being irrelevant. As a way to prepare for our adventure, I had decided to plant a garden. The June morning when Christopher left for his journalism fellowship, I got up at five a.m. to say good-bye, and subsequently could not fall back to sleep. Ordinarily, I am not an early riser; I love sleeping in on the weekends, and on school days I hit the snooze button repeatedly. But on this day, I had a plan. When we bought our house, I was excited that the backyard had two little raised garden beds, and I had resolved to start gardening as soon as we moved in. Of course, it was a year later on that early morning when I actually started digging. After extracting a promise from Christopher that he would call me when he arrived, I kissed him good-bye, threw on some old clothes, and went to work.

I spent the morning chopping at the rock-hard dirt and pulling weeds. I got to the gardening store just after they opened, and filled my cart with the makings of a vegetable garden: tomatoes, lettuce, bell peppers, jalapeños, and squash. I treated myself to a pair of gloves and a silly gardening hat. I justified the hat by claiming I needed it to protect my easily sunburned skin, but in reality I thought I might be a better gardener if I looked the part. Over the week I made several trips because I either needed more compost or realized I had more room and might be able to fit in one more tomato plant.

The garden didn't last long. By the time we were ready to start our dollar-a-day project, all that was left were some anemic, withered cherry tomatoes. Our dogs caused its untimely demise. They ate the jalapeños first; I found the peppers chewed up and spit out on the patio. The next day, Viola pulled the plant out of the ground, perhaps as retaliation for its spiciness. The lettuce I planted from seed didn't even have a chance to sprout; the day after I planted it, there was a large hole in the bed. My mom came to visit and we planted onions, which were ripped up one at a time over the course of the week. We laughed, but I was saddened each time the dogs came in with my labor on their breath. By the time Christopher got home, I was down to two bell pepper plants, three squash, and five tomatoes, which I think were spared due to the wire cages surrounding them. "You planted a salad bar for the dogs," became his running joke.

School began during the last week of August, and we were going to start our experiment that following week. We spent most of our first weekend running around to stores looking for the best prices, burning a few gallons of gas trekking around town. Finally, we ended up doing most of our shopping at Smart and Final. This fluorescent-lit industrial-style wholesaler was a far cry from our airy, eco-friendly natural food store. But at that time, they had the best prices for what we were doing. The price of beans per pound was cheaper than at the dollar store, but we would have to buy in much larger quantities. We thought we would be able to get more variety, but it was harder than we originally planned. We calculated the cost of our meals by adding up the prices of the ingredients for each meal and dividing it by the number of servings. The cheapest way to get the ingredient costs low was to buy in bulk.

We walked around using our phones as calculators, trying to find the best deals. Should we get fifteen pounds of flour, or twenty-five? Was it better to get pinto beans or black beans? Could we get both? Our shopping trip lasted much longer than our weekly visit to the store, and there were several times when we had to resignedly put items in the cart back on the shelf. In the end, we were surprised by what we couldn't get. It would have been roughly twenty-five cents per serving to buy black beans, but approximately eleven cents per serving for pinto beans. We could have bought a bag of ten apples for $2.99, but that made each apple $.29, and we decided it might not be worth it to use 29 percent of our daily allowance on a piece of fruit smaller than my fist. We bought white flour and wheat flour, but the wheat flour was a bleached blend, which meant that it was more difficult to get a good consistency for the seitan that we would be making. (Seitan is a low-cost meat alternative made from wheat flour.) We bought a twenty-pound bag of rice, jars of peanut butter and jelly, and a large bag of yeast for making our own bread, as well as several other industrial-sized items. The can of tomato sauce was so big we had to use both hands to carry it.

We then headed back to Jimbo's to buy a few items from the bulk bins. It ended up being less expensive per pound to buy oatmeal, popcorn, and dried garbanzo beans there. Overall, for the cheapest price per pound, our dollar store did not have the best bargains, and its proximity to Rico's made it a reminder of what we couldn't have. We were lucky that the dollar store had recently introduced a small produce display; it was an unlikely addition to the aisles lined with third-party brands and cheap household items, but we found some deals. They had onions, four for a dollar, and one of my favorite purchases: eight bulbs of garlic for a buck. We also got a one-pound bag of frozen broccoli. In total, we spent about eighty-five dollars during our first day of shopping. That was more than the total cost of what we would eat for the month (sixty dollars), but our idea was to calculate what we ate, not to eat every ounce we bought.

The rest of the afternoon was filled with opening huge bags, filling large green construction buckets with bulk foods, measuring and weighing the food, and starting meals for the week. We weighed every item to find out the cost, and we bought a food scale to make sure we were as accurate as possible. If a twenty-five-pound bag of pinto beans was $12.75, then two cups, weighing one pound, would cost approximately $.51. We used masking tape and a Sharpie to label the bright orange lid of each container with the cost per cup or teaspoon, depending on the item. Once everything was labeled, I started preparing a few things from our menu, including a batch of homemade seitan steaks and a loaf of bread. I put garbanzo and pinto beans in water so they could soak overnight before I cooked them the next day. As our first under-a-dollar meal came together, our excitement began to grow. This was going to be an adventure.

"HEY, WE'RE GOING to write a blog," Christopher said, the day before we started our project.

"Excuse me?" I replied. I was elbow deep in beans and flour. "I don't want to blog. I have nothing to say."

"Of course you do. Besides, I'm setting up our site, we just need to take a picture." He brought his laptop into the kitchen to show me what he had been working on while I toiled away making sure we would have food the following morning. The fact that he sprung the blog idea on me at the last minute might have worked to our benefit. Had I spent the entire summer thinking about the fact that I would be writing about my daily experiences for anyone to read, I would have vetoed it.

"Okay, fine," I agreed. I had gone along with everything else, so there seemed to be no harm in adding one more thing. "But can I shower and brush my hair before you post my picture on the Internet?"

The original intent of the blog was to share our experiences with our friends and family. Our families and Christopher's students became our first audience. When we set out, we didn't have a political agenda. Even though the idea came from the fact that there are people who have to eat on tight budgets, we weren't trying to make a statement. We didn't have something to prove. The only objective was that we make it through the month. When we prepared for the temporary change in our lifestyle, we weren't trying to show the way that people in poverty can, do, or should live; we were only trying to learn how we could eat for less. We knew that many people on stringent food budgets don't have the ability to price-check several stores, buy in bulk at the start of the month, transport and store large amounts of food, or have the time or means to cook everything from scratch. However, if we could explore these issues, we'd be happy to learn from it.

On that final night in August, we had our last dinner without worrying about the cost. We didn't go crazy or eat until we were sick, but instead we dined on what would soon become one of our staple meals: beans, rice, and tortillas. However, that night we savored the creamy Sour Supreme (a sour cream alternative), crunchy lettuce, juicy tomatoes, and spicy salsa. We ate this way so we would feel more prepared for the next day, but nothing could have prepared us for what we would experience in the next month.

And So It Begins

Christopher

It was still dark when I woke up, and the smell of fresh-baked bread filled the house. We had set the bread machine on a timer the night before. Kerri lay there with our old grumpy kitty, Mrs. B. (the *B* often takes on several meanings), sitting on her belly, calling out for breakfast. We have an alarm clock, but there is no need for it. When the missus is ready to eat, it's time to get up. I rolled out of bed, doing my best to get back into the routine for the new school year.

As Kerri started getting dressed, I began packing our lunches and preparing breakfast. Six cents' worth of rolled oats was thickening on the stove as I scooped one tablespoon of peanut butter and one tablespoon of jelly onto each slice of our homemade bread for our lunches. I popped some popcorn, salted it, and put it into small containers. Our lunches were looking much slimmer than usual, and I knew Kerri wouldn't be ecstatic over the thick mound of cooked oat groats, even if I put her portion in one of her favorite smiley face bowls. Kerri loved traveling in Scotland, but she didn't like this particular Scottish culinary tradition. While students at ancient universities in Scotland used to be released for "Meal Mondays" to collect more oats for food, this would not be a Monday treat she looked forward to. I was right. As Kerri took her first bite, her nose crinkled in disdain.

"If we split one tablespoon of margarine, it would only add three cents to the cost of breakfast," she said.

"Nah, let's skip it," I replied.

I picked up my briefcase and lighter-than-usual lunch bag and headed off to work. On the drive I thought to myself, "We can do this. It will be hard, and our meal options will be limited, but I'm optimistic." As I passed the manicured grass of the local park and took a right into the school parking lot, I considered what eating would be like in an emergency situation or natural disaster, and what would happen if the normal food system came to a sudden halt. I thought about all those zombie movies I loved, and how a group of survivalists often made the best of raw materials in the films. Now, this was not going to be the zombie apocalypse, but at least at the end of the month I would be better prepared just in case the walking dead actually did rise up and start to roam the earth. We would know what to do; we would survive.

At the beginning of my social justice class that day, I announced to my students that today was the beginning of our downsized culinary quest. They stared at me, confused and surprised. Some probably checked their schedules and considered switching into a class where the teacher might be a little more "normal." After ten seconds of awkward silence, hands started to sprout up all over the room. I smiled at the storm of questions from these high school seniors, most of whom had been raised with a magically replenishing fridge stocked full to bursting with all kinds of tasty treats. Their questions ranged from "What will you eat?" to suggestions like, "You should just get some twenty-nine-cent cheeseburgers at McDonald's and call it good." They didn't know that it had been over a decade since I stepped into the golden arches. Last time I checked, McDonald's offered little in the way of vegetarian fare. Surprisingly, snarky advice took a backseat as they mulled over the proposal. If there were any naysayers present, they kept quiet.

Within minutes, my students started thinking of all the ways we could get free or low-cost food. To my surprise, I had a room full of new allies. They suggested foraging the samples at wholesale stores like Costco on the weekends, and even tracking down some fresh fruit that was growing in various parts of the surrounding community. One girl drew me a map to the places where oranges were waiting to be picked. After class, she stayed behind and asked me if I'd be willing to tell her where the best deals on food were. I could see in her eyes that she *needed* to know, not because of some quaint curiosity about our efforts, but because her family had been struggling to figure out how to make it through the economic downturn. She told me that her family of four had about fifty dollars a week to spend on food. Our conversation took place just before the reports about the possibility of a recession began to emerge. She was a living, breathing early indicator that our country was headed for a financial maelstrom. I promised her that I would share anything that I could. We would hear more of these stories as our fledgling blog, intended for friends, family, and colleagues, gained more readers.

We knew before we started this project that while eating for less was a compelling challenge for us, for some people, it was a daily struggle. Kerri and I are both very aware of the amount of privilege that we were born into; we are lucky. Like the majority of our students, we were born white, middle or upper-middle class, and were fortunate enough to grow up without any major financial struggles. Our parents had jobs that allowed them to provide for us, and at times treat us with trips to Disneyland and weekend baseball games. Kerri's parents were both schoolteachers. My mom became a teacher after my parents divorced, and my father owned a successful small business. It was this recognition of our privileges that prompted me to start a place on our blog where people could sponsor our efforts. At the end of the project, we would donate all the money we had collected online to a local group that helps those who actually do struggle to find enough to eat. We eventually decided on an organization in Encinitas called the Community Resource Center, a group that provides social services for over ten thousand people a year, including services related to hunger. We chose this organization because of their focus on helping people become self-sufficient, and because we saw them making a palpable difference within our community.

This part of the project was an opportunity to do something that would actually help other people. Plus, we knew that our friends and family were economically stable enough to help others, and this was a way to bring that opportunity to them.

For the rest of the school day, I stayed busy. The morsels I had packed for lunch seemed to be just enough to get me through. The first few weeks of school are so hectic that sometimes it is easy to forget to eat altogether. Many of us eat rushed lunches, often while we push past hordes of students on our way to the copy room. The journey is often a failed mission, as the copiers resemble mechanical paper-spitting dragons. I have seen too many downtrodden teachers leave with only toner-covered hands to show for their courage. The typical teacher workday at the beginning of the school year makes Wall Street traders look like beach bums, and eating is often an afterthought. However, our lunchtime challenges were changing. Instead of struggling to find the time to eat, Kerri and I would eat little, and find it hard to maintain our energy levels.

Our first dinner was the same as the previous night: beans, rice, and tortillas. Kerri seemed to have survived the first day, but something was missing.

"That wasn't too bad," I said.

"No, it wasn't. I'm still a little hungry though," Kerri answered.

"Some of my students said there are orange trees near the school. I was thinking I'd drive by and check it out."

"That would be awesome. I could eat an orange right about now."

We sat looking at each other. It was clear that we both needed just a little more to eat. It could have been psychological, but we were itching for something to top off our first day. We had each spent ninety-one cents for our meals throughout the day, and that remaining nine cents was burning a hole in our stomachs. My sweet tooth would have to find a way to survive this month without chocolate.

As I stared into the open cupboards, wondering where to expend these last few pennies, it dawned on me: peanut butter. For six cents a tablespoon, this plastic tub of high-fructose corn syrup–sweetened goodness was the shining light in the darkness of our barren pantry.

I called to Kerri, "You want a tablespoon of peanut butter?" She came into the kitchen with a smile on her face; she didn't need to say a word. I took the tablespoon off the drying rack and scooped out one serving for each of us—a habit I picked up from watching my father dig into jars of peanut butter when I was a kid. I put the spoon in my mouth and savored it. The salty sweetness opened my salivary floodgates, and I could feel the smooth butter move around in my mouth. I made it last for as long as I could, and licked the spoon clean. Nothing could be wasted. This was the perfect reward for surviving the first day.

The next day the menu was the same, but my students came to class armed with new questions that led to some engaging discussions about poverty, local food pantries, and clever ways to raise the profile of other important issues. The student who had asked me about finding low-cost food stayed behind again, and we got to talking about the privilege of eating high-end natural foods. We then discussed how the remaining indigenous people on our planet sustain themselves. We were both left with questions about how the global food system got to the point it's at today.

During that second day, I felt more energized than usual. By the time I got home, I had two different messages from casting departments in Hollywood who were calling to offer me auditions: one for a game show and one for a reality TV show. I'm not an actor and have no aspirations to become one, but I love to put myself in new situations. I think it's good to experiment with situations, just to see what happens. I got to thinking about these new television opportunities during dinner. We sat there eagerly chomping away on our bean and rice burritos, and I imagined how funny it would be for my friends to see me, the vegan, appearing on a network program squeezed between Taco Bell and Burger King commercials.

Then I started thinking about how often we are told to eat. Television and radio commercials offer us $1.99 "Super Value" meals with fast-moving images of food set to snazzy music. The message is clear: EAT. Most of us in the United States eat three squares a day without really giving it a second thought. We are surrounded by an empire of cereals, sodas, and snacks. Colorful packages line the shelves of brightly lit big-box stores, each proclaiming how *healthy* its contents are. Most folks walk right past the fresh fruits and vegetables. Just eating a salad gives us a sense of holiness. People eat far more fats and sugars than the more nutritious food options. Unfortunately, when one looks at the number of new food products introduced into stores in combination with how large companies spend their marketing dollars, it becomes easy to see why our country is overweight. It should come as no surprise that only 2.2 percent of all food-marketing dollars are spent on fruits and vegetables, whereas 70 percent of advertising dollars are spent on convenience foods, candy and snacks, alcoholic beverages, soft drinks, and desserts.

Additionally, in a study conducted in 1998 that categorized the 11,037 new food products introduced that year, over 2,000 of them were candy, gum, and snacks, while only 375 were fruits and vegetables. Not only that, but citizens in our country have more food available to them than ever before. In her book *Food Politics*, Marion Nestle points to data from the United States Department of Agriculture, indicating that the U.S. food supply increased from 3,200 calories per capita in 1970 to 3,900 in the late 1990s. This means that in the United States, there is enough food for each of us to consume nearly twice what we need.

Meats, grains, and sweets are the most profitable products, which is why they constitute the lion's share of advertising dollars. They are also the cheapest calories on the market. In a study by researchers at the University of Washington, scientists spent two years comparing the costs of 370 products sold at Seattle supermarkets. They found that high-calorie, energy-dense foods cost on average only $1.76 per 1,000 calories, whereas low-energy, nutritious foods cost $18.16 for the same amount of calories. What is perhaps more striking is that the high-calorie foods dropped in price by 1.8 percent, whereas low-calorie foods like fruits and vegetables increased by 19.5 percent during the course of the study.

Now, there are some folks, like the people at the Heritage Foundation, a conservative think tank, who push the notion that it is not the industry's fault that people are eating more, and eating more of these high-calorie foods. They believe that it is up to the consumer to make the nutritional choices that are best for them. However, the less money you have, the less choice you have. Most people know that feeding kids a Happy Meal for dinner a few nights a week is not the best nutritional choice, but when that is the cheapest, most filling, and most accessible option, it's clear why it is also one of the most common.

During our experiment, we couldn't afford either fast food or most fruits and vegetables. I never knew how much I would miss my vegetables until I started this endeavor. My mind continued to spin when trying to comprehend the interconnection of all the issues. I thought about how a third of the children in the United States eat fast food every day. I thought about the obesity epidemic. I thought about the global paradox that over 800 million people on earth don't have enough to eat, yet in the developing world, over a billion people are overweight. Then I was struck by something more immediate: the realization that we would be eating the same foods for the rest of the month.

The idea of eating the same staple ingredients for weeks at a time was already beginning to feel daunting. Stumped, we did some brainstorming. We looked at Mexican, Chinese, and Indian cuisines for inspiration about how to avoid the mundane. These cuisines use some of the same basic ingredients and make a wide variety of dishes, and we were hoping for similar success. Yet, without bell peppers in our fajitas, or cauliflower in our aloo gobi, the next few weeks would be bleak.

Later that night, I checked our blog. We had received a few donations for the Community Resource Center from complete strangers. It wasn't a lot, but $135 by the second day wasn't a bad start, especially considering that we weren't advertising our project to anyone. We simply told some friends and our family members, and all of a sudden we were receiving e-mails and, better yet, money to give to our local center. If this turned out to be a way to help people, then it would be worth the sacrifice. After a less-than-filling dinner, I looked at Kerri, and she stared back.

"Are you thinking what I'm thinking?" she asked.

"Peanut butter?"

"Yeah."

"Definitely."

We tried for a moment to convince ourselves that this tablespoon of peanut butter was a good source of protein, which it generally is, but the truth was that it was the closest thing to dessert within our budget, and we craved it. It felt good to indulge in this small way.

When we woke the next morning, I remembered that it was Back to School Night, the single occasion all year when most parents come to the school to meet their students' teachers. I knew that it would be a late evening, so Kerri planned to come home relatively soon after school and cook one of the meals we had decided on the night before: chana masala. This Indian dish is simple: cooked garbanzo beans in a tomato-based sauce, mixed with spices like garam masala, turmeric, cumin, and paprika. It doesn't seem like much, but with rice, it can be quite filling. The thought of the evening meal propelled me through most of the day, but by the time parents started showing up at the school that evening, I was surprised to find that they, too, were wondering what I would be having for dinner.

During the ten minutes that teachers get with each batch of parents, I usually introduce myself and the goals of the course, then use the remainder of the time to answer questions. These questions usually cover a pretty wide range, as each parent has individual concerns about what the class will be like for his or her child. This year, things were different. By the time I got to the question and answer portion of my presentation, no one seemed to be worried about what their children would be learning. The first question came from a woman in the back of the room: "What's it like to eat on a dollar a day?"

I didn't expect to be answering questions about my diet in a room full of parents. So I did what most teachers do when they are caught off guard by an off-topic question from a student: I looked around the room. Before I could answer, a gentleman in the front row spoke. "Yeah, we heard all about this dollar-a-day thing. Tell us about it." Anxiously, I glanced around again and saw that parents were smiling and seemed to be genuinely interested. I began to speak.

"Well, it's just this project that my partner and I started a couple of days ago. We want to see if we can manage."

"How long are you going to do it?" shouted another parent in the back.

"For the rest of the month."

There was a collective gasp.

"What did you eat today?" a concerned mother asked.

I continued explaining our efforts for the remainder of our time together. Then, finally, the bell rang and I was saved. I thanked them for coming and reminded them to keep in contact with me throughout the year if they had any questions or concerns about their children. They lingered. I moved toward the door to signal that I was getting ready to meet the next group of parents, but several of them quickly approached me. Typically, at this point, some parents are eager to tell me about the individual needs of their kids. Tonight was different. Every conversation centered around our attempt to eat on a dollar a day. By the time they had all moved on to their students' next class, I took a deep breath and thought to myself, "That was weird." I hoped that the next class would be less inquisitive, but it wasn't. As the night carried on, it seemed that the word was out with parents, and first period was just the warning shot. It wasn't until the last group of the night, my journalism class, when things finally seemed to be winding down. Delaney, my student editor, led this session, but by the time she was done and we opened up for questions, the dollar diet had parents talking. I could only imagine the conversations in the cars of parents at the end of the night. Exhausted, I packed up and headed home.

As I walked in the door, I was tuckered out. It had been nine hours since I last ate, and the calories from my PB&J sandwich had been used up long ago. Kerri scooped some chana masala and rice onto plates, and I proceeded to recount the events of the night. She, too, was surprised by the parents' interest in our project. She told me about her day, and as we ate, we talked about the ways in which we had already started looking at our lives differently. Kerri said that it seemed contradictory to be eating on a dollar a day while brushing her teeth with five-dollar toothpaste. We realized how rarely we stop to think about all that we have. Beyond the material luxuries that we enjoy—living in our home, owning cars, being able to care for our pets—we thought about the safety of our community, the security of our jobs, and many of the other privileges that often go unconsidered in our daily lives.

Then Kerri brought up a conversation that she'd had earlier in the day with a friend. In addition to all of the other privileges we enjoy, we also had the liberty to buy fresh produce, and lots of it. Kerri reflected on how frustrating it is to consider that over 36 million people in our country don't have that same opportunity. Poor Americans are often unable to afford fresh produce. Some forgo it because, when given the option between an orange and a ninety-nine-cent taco, it is clear which one provides the most calories for the money. Others live in areas completely devoid of grocery stores. They don't have access to high quality food and are left to find sustenance in fast-food restaurants, since grocery chains are reticent to enter these areas. As this phenomenon predominantly occurs in areas populated by people of color, it has been called "food apartheid."

In his book *Stuffed & Starved*, Raj Patel outlines this "supermarket redlining," a term borrowed from the illegal practice of banks using a red pen to circle these neighborhoods and refusing to lend to anyone within them. Patel makes it clear that this practice leaves poor people of color destined for nutritional inadequacy and cites several studies that show that when healthy food becomes available, more fruits and vegetables are eaten.

Even more surprising is a study cited by Patel and conducted by New York City's Department of Consumer Affairs, where an 8.8 percent difference in prices was found between low-income neighborhoods and more affluent ones. Poorer areas were paying *more* than well-to-do areas for the same foods. As dinner ended, we felt thankful for all that we had, and upon calculating our daily totals, which hovered around ninety cents for the day, we smiled and grabbed the peanut butter.

Over the next few days, our new food life started to show some signs of wear. I began getting headaches at work, and at one point felt so light-headed that I had to hold on to my lectern for stability. Soon after, I went to the school nurse between classes to ask her if she had any recommendations. Diane is one of the most helpful and in-touch people I have ever met. Her warmth and willingness to help keep students healthy are unmatched, and I knew I could lean on her in this moment of desperation.

"Drink more water. That's what Gandhi did."

Now, I am not Gandhi, but it was sage advice. I started downing water like an elephant at a watering hole, and it worked. I felt better. However, my initial boost of energy from the first two days had all but disappeared. I would come home and have to refrain from gorging myself on anything in sight. Days at work seemed longer, and by the end of the first week, I felt utterly exhausted. I wasn't alone. That Friday, Kerri and I made the drive to Hollywood for one of my auditions. We left right after school got out, and within twenty minutes, Kerri fell asleep in the passenger seat. On the drive home, she put in a call to her mom to tell her about our experience at the lot where they shoot the TV show *Heroes* and one of our favorites, *Dexter*. Kerri's mom was more interested in our health than the audition. She worried that we would become deficient in vitamin C and develop scurvy. Neither one of us had actually considered the possibility. Scurvy? Wasn't that something that pirates got back in the olden days by staying out too long at sea? Her concern forced us to think about the possibility that we could actually hurt our bodies by doing this project, but we wanted to forge ahead.

The next morning I stepped onto the scale in our bathroom. In one week, I had already lost four pounds. Upon entering the kitchen, I could see that Kerri was also worried. She had foraged a lemon from our front yard and dropped a couple of slices in her water. I told her about my weight loss, and she admitted that she, too, had been thinking about her own half-pound fluctuations.

While we were both tired, we knew that the rest of our worries were probably psychological. Kerri had been staying late at work with the debate team, which she coaches, and the first few weeks of a new school year are always trying. We were paying extra attention to the way our bodies were reacting because we had made a significant change in diet. Prior to this challenge, we would feast on mountains of food, and now the meager portions on our small plates never looked like enough. Beyond that, we had started to get snippy with each other around dinnertime. Taking out the ingredients and setting them on the counter, I could see the resentment on Kerri's face. This was a chore. The sounds of clanging cookware echoed the frustration in the room as the dogs ducked their heads and recoiled from our angst. Between calculating the costs of each individual ingredient and the pressure on Kerri to cook dinner after being at work all day, it helped to slam cupboard doors. No one wants to come home to housework after working all day, and my unwillingness to help was that of a prototypical teenager at odds with his or her parents. If Kerri asked me to do something, I sighed with obvious irritation. We ate dinner in relative silence. The next morning, we made up for lost energy by sleeping late and missing breakfast, but on Sunday I was determined to make up for two days of stress and exasperation.

I love breakfast foods, which is why I often put together our weekend morning meals. French toast, pancakes, waffles, hash browns—you name it and I've made it for breakfast at one point or another. When I awoke on Sunday, I was determined to celebrate our first week by taking a break from our drab oatmeal regimen and surprising Kerri with a pancake breakfast. After she had spent most evenings putting together our dinners, I needed to show her how much I appreciated her efforts. Plus, I knew that she was still bitter about the broccoli. On our first shopping trip we had picked up a one-pound bag of frozen broccoli at the dollar store; it was a great find. When we opened it, to our dismay, it was all pale green stems and one limp floret. Talk about false advertising. We couldn't help but chuckle at our own anticipation. When Kerri portioned out our meal, she cut the tiny floret in half so that we each got some of the "good" part. The spoonful of peanut butter for dessert wasn't enough to make up for the disappointment.

So that morning I felt compelled to go out of my way to make sure that she would at least enjoy breakfast. I went to the shelf, grabbed a cookbook, opened up to the pancake recipe, and started doing the math to see how much it would cost. If I got six pancakes out of the batch, they would come to five cents each. The only challenge would be getting some syrup. I sat there wondering how I could do this.

Then it struck me. Our "rules" stated that if something was free to everyone in our area, then we could eat it without charge. I didn't even bother with shoes. I slipped on my sandals, donned a hooded sweatshirt, hopped in the car, and headed to a place I hadn't been to in over a decade: McDonald's. Fast-food joints had all kinds of free condiments, and in the mornings, syrup was one of them. I pulled open the doors and swerved past the seniors to the counter, on a mission. Before the woman behind the register could welcome me, I stated my case.

"Can I get some syrup?"

She didn't even flinch. She made her way to the supply hiding under another part of the counter, pulled out two packages, and dropped them in my outstretched hand. The small plastic tubs were warm in my palm. Victory was mine. I would be able to wake Kerri to a delicious breakfast that would give her the motivation to keep going.

Before I pulled out of the parking lot to head for home, I thought about how easy that was. I wondered if I could do it again at the Burger King down the street; it was worth a shot. If I could acquire a little more I'd be able to save some for next weekend. Ten minutes later I burst out of Burger King's doors with two more servings of sweet magic. I felt like a king but probably looked more like Gollum protecting his "precious" as I smiled in selfish joy. I was on a roll. I looked down at my passenger seat and saw the map that one of my students had drawn for me earlier in the week. If X marked the spot, it wouldn't be long before I was harvesting some community oranges that lined the street near a housing development behind my work. My engine purred and the roads cleared to make way for me.

Of course, no quest would be complete without some type of tribulation. After I had driven up and down the streets of identical tract homes, I started to become discouraged. I had seen plenty of lemons, but no oranges. Had my student misled me? Did she know the difference between oranges and lemons? How could I keep driving slowly through the pristine suburbs without alerting the neighborhood watch? Looking for fruit trees on the side of the road while driving isn't exactly the safest of enterprises, but I could already taste the fresh-squeezed orange juice, and I wasn't about to give up. Little did I know that my search was in vain, and close to an hour later I relented. Disappointed by my "fruitless" search, I clutched the syrup packages and remembered to be thankful for what I had.

Kerri loved the pancakes, mainly because she didn't have to eat oatmeal, and I felt good about that. Later that day I would forage a lollipop at a local tattoo parlor, and even though Kerri felt that I was breaking one of our rules, I sat there enjoying the second rush of sugar on my palate. Of course, this didn't stop us from eating our habitual tablespoon of peanut butter goodness later that evening.

At around three a.m., something wasn't right. While I had been riding high on the wave of free sugar from earlier in the day, my bowels wouldn't let me sleep. I wasn't sure if it was the no-cheese pizza that I made for dinner, or just my system in shock, but either way, I was paying for it now. I was frightened that I had become sick, and I worried that there was no way I would be ready for work a few hours from now. I started to think that maybe this dollar thing wasn't worth it.

The Cookie War

Kerri

On Monday, just one week after we had started this project, I walked through the door with my arms full of papers to grade, despite the futility of bringing them home. Like many of my colleagues, I have a terrible habit of taking student papers on a "field trip," a teaching term that means taking work home and then bringing it back the next day without having graded anything. I do this at least once a week. I have good intentions, but by the time I get home, I've been working for ten to twelve hours and don't want to do anything but spend time with Christopher and the kids—our dogs, Viola and Horatio, and Mrs. B., our perpetually perturbed cat. This night was no different. When I stepped inside, Christopher was waiting for me with the dogs close at his heels. They had me surrounded.

"Hi," he said, smiling, as he took my bags and papers from my hands. "I need you to do something for me." I didn't trust his smile; it seemed like he was up to something.

"Can I have a minute to walk in the door?"

"Nope, I need you to hold this for me so I can take a picture."

I didn't want my picture taken. I had been at work late that night; Christopher had dinner-making duty so that we could eat as soon as

I got home. The long day had left me exhausted, and I needed to eat dinner and take a shower to wash the twelve hours of high school off my skin. Next thing I knew, a handwritten sign and a wooden spoon were thrust into my hands. Christopher moved me into the light and told me to smile. I played along. After all, he had gone out of his way for me that weekend to make pancakes. Besides, I knew that food would come sooner if I complied. I gave my best take-the-damn-picture-so-I-can-eat-or-I-may-kill-you smile, and the camera clicked away.

I still didn't know what had gotten into him. It seemed as if inspiration struck my otherwise rational partner while he prepared our forty-cent serving of beans and rice, which had been getting cold on the stove as we fretted over the pictures. The sign I held proclaimed September 8 "National Beans and Rice Day." Christopher hoped that it would catch on. He wanted it to be a day when we would "celebrate the simple beauty in a mound of rice and the delicate texture of a pile of beans, so that all who come after us will know how seriously we take our food." I laughed at his excitement about his new national holiday; maybe it was the lack of food or the delirium from spending too much time at work that contributed to the giddiness. We started that week energized, but we didn't know that a gritty battle of the wills would ensue.

By Wednesday, it became apparent that the novelty of our project would not last much longer, at least not for me. So far our blog had attracted a few more readers than we had planned. We figured that our parents and friends would read it, but others had found us and were following our journey as well. Friends and coworkers of our friends and family were now also reading. Christopher's mom's fifth-grade health class was reading it, too. I knew that if people were interested in what we were doing, then I would have to keep going, but I felt myself starting to struggle with the regimen. I wanted more food than the diet allowed; it consumed my thoughts. I wanted a burrito. A warm tortilla holding not just some beans and rice, but chock-full of lettuce, tomato, and avocado prepared in the hands of a professional, someone who knows how to fill the tortilla almost to its bursting point and then lovingly wrap it so that nothing will slip out. I wanted to drench it in salsa and savor my side of extra crispy French fries.

Since the meager dollar-a-day portions didn't satiate my hunger, food became the focus of my existence. When we weren't preparing food, we were eating. When we weren't eating, we were thinking about eating. It became increasingly impossible to ignore the abundance of food surrounding me, and the fact that I couldn't have it. Not only that, but I began focusing on the amount of food I saw wasted. It seemed that every day I saw people throwing away perfectly good food. For us, waste wasn't an option. Everything was accounted for; every grain of rice and every pinto bean had a price tag. No longer did I toss the scraps of our food to the dogs while I cooked. Every night they followed me around the kitchen, tails wagging in hope that I would drop something, but I was vigilant. We precisely measured out every bite, and we not only appreciated the food that we had, we cringed at the idea of something going to waste.

I saw the most waste at school. I winced when I witnessed sandwiches tossed away, half-full bags of chips pushed by the wind across the campus, and once-bitten apples left in the quad to rot. One of my students habitually throws unopened granola bars and bags of chips into the trash if they aren't the flavors he likes. I wondered if his parents had any idea that their son threw away the food they worked hard to provide. I thought about whether this was a consequence of the largely affluent area where I teach, or just the way teenagers take food for granted. But the waste didn't stop with the students.

At our midweek staff meeting during the second week of school, the administration provided lunch, and my coworker Dave sat at my table with his taco, chips, and salsa. My recollection of the meeting is hazy, but I can still remember the smell of the salsa. I spent half of the meeting drooling and trying to use my telepathic powers to get him to eat the last few bites so I wouldn't have to look at it anymore. The voices of administrators, eerily reminiscent of the "waah waah waah" of Charlie Brown's teachers, droned on in the background. Their announcements became indecipherable, and their mandates landed nowhere near my consciousness. I focused on the food languishing on Dave's plate. For the first time, I considered breaking the rules. I didn't entertain the thought for long, but it took all of my willpower to not reach over and snag a chip. Walking back to my classroom, I couldn't help but wonder what would become of the leftover trays of Mexican food. I hoped that someone would have the decency to pack up the rice and add it to a homemade soup. I imagined the beans being plopped into reusable containers and carried home as side dishes for dinner. I envied the person lucky enough to sequester the salsa and use it later. There is a reason why salsa has surpassed ketchup as America's number one condiment; never before had I felt such food envy. The idea that Wednesday's lunch could become Thursday's trash left me feeling disgusted. I realized that I would have to start spending more of my lunches working alone in my classroom so I wouldn't be surrounded by people wasting perfectly good food. Our rules said we could have free food only if it was available to everyone. If this free food hadn't been limited to my school's staff, I would have eaten my fill, then hovered around after lunch to see what I could take home.

Before this point, I had only a cursory understanding of how much food I wasted. Like many people, I don't like to be wasteful, but I get squeamish if I think that food is "old" or has been in the refrigerator for more than a few days. Despite my queasiness, I always feel compelled to bring home restaurant leftovers, and with few exceptions, I let them sit in the refrigerator until Christopher eats them, or until they actually do spoil and need to be thrown out. Christopher, on the other hand, seems convinced that food cannot go bad. To me, four days is the limit for homemade leftovers; with no logical reasoning to support this, two days is the maximum for restaurant food. On the other hand, Christopher's "method" for a food safety check is much more lax. Regardless of how long the item has been lurking in the back corners of the fridge, his process involves opening the container, smelling the contents, and then pronouncing them edible; if it's questionable, he'll dip in a finger and taste it. If the leftover passes muster on both the smell and the taste tests, Christopher will not only eat it, but also gladly serve it to others. We continue to disagree on this level of quality control, probably because we've had far different experiences with what can be considered edible.

Before we met, Christopher volunteered for a while with an organization called Food Not Bombs that works to feed the hungry with the excess food disposed of daily by the food industry. While living in the San Francisco Bay Area, Christopher was brought into the fold by one of his college roommates. This revolutionary movement, started in Massachusetts in 1980 by an anti-nuclear activist, grew into a worldwide phenomenon that has hundreds of autonomous chapters operating throughout the Americas, Europe, Africa, the Middle East, Asia, and Australia. Without a headquarters, formal leadership, or support from major media outlets, Food Not Bombs has many victories worth mentioning. It was the only organization in San Francisco providing hot meals to the survivors of the 1989 earthquake. They were also the first to provide hot meals for rescue workers responding to the September 11 World Trade Center attacks, and its volunteers were among the first to provide food and help to the survivors of the Asian tsunami and Hurricane Katrina. Food Not Bombs is now working to help those most affected by the recession in the United States by organizing Food Not Lawns community gardens and housing the homeless with splinter activities like Homes Not Jails. This movement to end war and poverty has no formal leaders, and since its inception has also spawned other groups like Bikes Not Bombs, which collects and repairs used bicycles to provide to people in low-income communities. The members of this grassroots movement come from all sorts of different activist networks; many work on poverty issues, animal rights issues, and environmental sustainability projects. The strength of Food Not Bombs, like any group, lies in its diversity, and for Christopher, it helped him see food waste firsthand. His time spent turning "waste" into hot vegetarian meals gave him a broader sense of what was edible.

My outlook on waste was shaped by a different experience. The six and a half years I spent working in a grocery store taught me that the "sell-by" date is just that: the last day an item can be *sold*. In all reality, depending on the item, it may not spoil for another week. In fact, in early 2009, as people were becoming more economically strained, there were reports of the growing popularity of grocery store auctions, where people thronged to bid on food that had reached its sell-by date. Yet regardless of knowing that food would last a little longer, at home I still tossed out anything that reached its date.

Almost all members of my family have worked in a grocery store at some point in their lives. My grandfather owned his own store for a few years before going to work for a friend who was starting a chain in northern California. He worked for the company for thirty-two years, and much of my family has worked in stores for the chain. Because of this, I've always had the idea that if food looks suspicious or you can't remember when you bought it, you should throw it out and buy a replacement. Food has never made me ill, but I worry that the day after the expiration date, food suddenly goes bad. A few years ago I told my mom this and she said, "I think you get that from me." She has the same fear and would rather run to the store than take the risk.

In addition, I'd never had to wonder when or if I would be getting my next meal, so I'd never really considered what I was wasting. I thought nothing of letting vegetables rot in the refrigerator or tossing some item out because it might be bad. When I worked at the grocery store, it was convenient to just buy what I needed for a meal before I left work. While my coworkers pulled items off the shelves, people like Christopher waited out back to get knee deep in the Dumpster, searching for the lost treasures of a system built on product throughput. Of course, the store I worked for locked its Dumpsters. The rationale, I believe, was that they did not want to be held responsible if someone ate spoiled food and became ill. In high school, I worked at a movie theater, and every night the closing concession worker filled large garbage bags with the leftover popcorn and threw it away. Even if an employee or customer asked, they would not be allowed to take any home; it was against policy. In order to protect themselves, many companies throw out perfectly good food every day.

Once I was back in my classroom after the meeting, I started to realize the absurdity of my past fears concerning leftover food. I had thrown away too much food in my lifetime, and I could now see the wastefulness of my actions. I needed to change. My perception was shifting. My concept of "good" and "bad" food had to evolve if we were going to make it two more weeks on a dollar each a day. Even if something was past its prime, I would eat it.

The next morning when I walked onto campus, I saw an apple lying in the dirt. From my viewpoint, it appeared that the apple had not yet been bitten. I seriously considered going back to pick it up and stow it away for later, but I was too much of a wimp. Later that day I saw one of my students throwing away cucumber sticks and cherry tomatoes. I wanted to stop her, but I could imagine the conversation with the principal, or her parents, about why I had to beg students for their leftovers. I envisioned rumors spreading around campus about how Ms. Leonard rummaged for food in the trash cans after lunch. The reality is that people tend to waste food when there is an abundance of it, not when there is a limited supply. While I faced this issue at school, Christopher faced similar circumstances at meetings off campus.

Christopher would be traveling to East Africa with Rotary International in January; he had applied for the fellowship and was one of five San Diego county teachers selected. They required that he attend a few meetings before leaving, and all of these meetings were scheduled around meals. On the morning of our thirteenth day, he attended the district conference at the Salk Institute in La Jolla. The breakfast did not disappoint the grumbling tummies of Rotary members, but it overwhelmed Christopher. Trays piled high with fresh melon, strawberries, and standard American diet staples like eggs, bacon, and toast lined the walls. Both of our meetings made us realize the abundance of free food that we have access to, and that these opportunities for free food occur more often than we had previously thought. Again, the food wasn't available to everyone, only to the members of the Rotary club and their guests, so it didn't fall into our "free" category.

Our meetings weren't the only places where we encountered the abundance of food offered to select groups of people. We like to attend lectures at the universities in our area, which almost always have cookie trays with coffee and tea. Some offer such a wide variety of catered appetizers that it seemed everyone in attendance could have had a full meal. But it doesn't stop there. At least a few times a year, lunch is provided to us at staff meetings. At my school, the parent organization does a wonderful job of making sure that teachers know they are appreciated. We get breakfast served at the start of the year, on holidays, on teacher appreciation day, and at the end of the year, as well. The parents provide sandwiches for Back to School Night so we don't have to rush home and back in the short time between school and the evening program; many teachers would skip dinner altogether if not for the parents' generosity. My Associated Student Body sponsors "Teacher Javas" two or three times a year, where they have coffee, bagels, and fruit for teachers in the morning. Obviously, this isn't the case in most jobs.

When I worked at the movie theater, we could have all the popcorn and soda we wanted during our breaks. I couldn't begin to calculate how much popcorn I consumed that year, but this minimum wage job never provided meals or snacks for meetings. When we are concerned about where our next meal is coming from, we pause before tossing away leftovers. When we know there is a limited amount, we ration and carefully measure. In third-world countries, and in the homes of America's poor, this is usually true. Waste is not an option. But for most Americans, we live in the land of cheap food.

This level of abundance is in part due to the fact, as Michael Pollan and others have pointed out, that most Americans are eating foods made from corn and soy. Even when you think you're drinking something as simple as lemonade, you're bound to be drinking syrup made from corn. If you pick up a hamburger at the drive-through, the cow you are about to eat spent nearly its entire existence eating corn, which is not what they evolved to eat. And the bun that is now home to the dead cow in your grasp most likely is sweetened with corn. Not to mention the ketchup you top it with, and the soda that helps you wash it down. All include corn.

Before becoming vegan, I never looked at the ingredients labels of what I was eating unless I was wondering about the calorie count. Once I started taking a more active interest in what I was consuming, I found that in many packaged foods there seems to be an abundance of ingredients that come from a laboratory instead of from the soil. Not only that, but most foods I was eating contained corn in some form or another. According to the USDA, the United States plants eighty million acres of corn. The abundance of this product makes it an inexpensive item that it seems can be added to anything. At least this new meal plan limited our intake of Iowa's cash crop and America's superfood—kind of. The peanut butter we had been treating ourselves with and the jelly on our sandwiches both listed high-fructose corn syrup as one of the top ingredients. Because this food is comparatively cheap, we tend not to think as much about tossing it out. Only when there is abundance do we waste.

Despite the plenty surrounding us, by Friday of the second week the physical and emotional impacts of our dollar-diet had become more apparent. I had lost three pounds, and Christopher had shed seven. So far, my lunches were getting me through the school day, but eating on a dollar a day leaves little economic room for those afternoon snacks that keep me going until dinnertime, and on days I stayed late, I needed something more. Since I started teaching four years ago, I have been the school's debate coach. It is a time-consuming commitment, and that's putting it lightly. After those first three weeks of school, I already had several twelve-hour days under my belt; at least three were meetings with debate parents to let them know what was in store and to teach them how to judge at our tournaments. This was on top of staying after school for meetings with students. I hadn't told my students about our dollar project, so there was no discussion of eating at my Back to School Night, only of how my classes would run; it was far different from Christopher's evening the week before. In addition, I would be hosting and running our league's first debate tournament of the year that coming weekend. Just the idea of this weekend-long event made me tired. I was drained and hungry, which in combination can make anyone cranky.

EARLIER IN THE week, one of my English classes had somehow started discussing oatmeal. I lamented that I had been eating the gloppy substance plain for two weeks, and at this point the conversation turned to oatmeal cookies. A few students were appalled that I didn't care for them. The next day a student brought me a cookie that he had made. I took it, but I didn't eat it. At that point I still felt strong. Later in the week it was a different story.

Friday was the first debate tournament of the year, and my school was the host. By the end of the last period, I was frantically running around. I needed to make sure the classroom doors were unlocked, judges were in place, visiting teams knew where to go, and the first round was matched and ready to post. Then, two of my first-year debaters showed up with two plates full of vegan chocolate chip cookies—one to sell at concessions, and one for the coaches. So began the Great Cookie War.

As I worked through the evening, I tried to ignore the plate. Friday nights used to be a time to see friends, go to the movies, or relax after a hard workweek, but upon becoming a debate team coach, I worked Friday night and all day Saturday. On that evening, I paid attention to my tasks and tried not to notice as other coaches walked by and grabbed a cookie without even thinking about it. But those cookies were all I could think about.

During the second round of events, I sneaked outside to call Christopher. I let the darkness envelop me as I punched in the number. The conversation started out playfully. I presented my plan: I would eat one cookie, or maybe just a half, but I would buy it from concessions and calculate the fifty-cent cost into my food total for the day. I thought my logic was sound, my case clear, and my motives pure. Christopher replied that to eat this cookie was breaking a rule. I tried a new tactic: I argued that we said we could eat food that was free to anyone. I pointed out that judges and coaches eat for free at tournaments, and we welcomed anyone to come and judge. In fact, we often begged people to come. He said that it was unlikely that a person unaffiliated with the school or the event would come onto campus to get free food. I countered that their purpose for coming to campus didn't matter, but rather that they *could*. He said that this wasn't a reasonable assumption. Nearing exasperation, I upped the stakes. I reminded him that just a few days before, he ate a "free" sucker from a jar in a tattoo parlor. I felt that it was much more likely for someone to see an event happening at a school and wander by to graze some food than it was for someone to walk into a tattoo parlor to get a lollipop. He failed to see my logic.

That was it: I had to fight dirty. I told him that he had bent the rules and justified it for his own benefit, but was now going out of his way to make me feel guilty for wanting to eat a cookie that I was willing to pay for. I told him that he had cheated, yet he was denying me a cookie because he wasn't there to have one. He claimed that I would have to find out all of the ingredients and calculate the cost per cookie in order for it to work. But that was ridiculous; we didn't charge ourselves for the individual ingredients in the ramen noodles or spaghetti that we had purchased. I felt that prepared foods were different; he insisted that this would violate our rules.

By this point, I was furious, far more so than anyone should ever get over a cookie. While most couples were at home watching a movie, or out with friends, I was standing in the dark, still at work, surrounded by hundreds of students, many of whom were debating the topic of whether or not the federal government should increase subsidies for alternative energy—while I, the crazy woman running this thing, was debating my partner over a cookie. As the second rounds came to an end, I had to make a decision: continue the argument, or get back to work. I hung up, trying not to cry. Like any other couple, Christopher and I have disagreements, but usually they don't last long. I don't think I have ever been as angry with him as I was at that moment. Images of going home and packing up my belongings flashed through my mind. How could I stay with some-one who would give me such grief over a cookie?

The answer came later that night. I spent the evening fuming; it took a great effort to keep the tournament going while I waited for Christopher to bring me dinner as we had planned. He showed up late, and that added to my frustration. He arrived at around eight thirty, and I hadn't eaten since noon. He came over to where I sat in a student desk surrounded by schedules and results. The other coaches huddled around the plate of cookies, chatting, unaware of the misery caused by those tiny morsels. Christopher approached.

"I'm sorry," he said.

Instantly my anger dissipated and I wrapped my arms around him, noticing that he felt thinner. I apologized as well, and he set my dinner down. He brought me beans, rice, and tortillas, with the added treat of fried potatoes. Then he reminded me why I fell in love with him: He handed me two homemade peanut butter cookies. He was late bringing me dinner not because he was angry, but be-cause he had spent time finding a cookie recipe that we could afford.

Vegetable Liberation

Christopher

Pulling into the crowded parking lot, I wondered if people who struggled financially shopped at places like this. Mostly white families pushed SUV-sized carts through the Costco entrance as an employee checked for their membership cards. I pulled mine from my wallet to signal that I had paid my dues; I belonged. Kerri and I weren't sure if we would actually buy anything that day, but two weeks without fresh produce had made us desperate. Pushing the cart toward the back of the store, I thought about the large bags of carrots, cartons of blueberries, and other industrial-sized servings of plant life that could become part of our meals. I longed for the crunch of vegetables between my teeth, the bitter taste of a bell pepper, the vapid flavor of romaine lettuce. I needed my veggies, and I needed them now.

Deftly I maneuvered around whining children and their parents. I hung a left at the DVDs and barreled down the aisle of leftover beach towels. Kerri and my sister, Heather, who'd come along to observe how we shopped on our dollar experiment, did their best to keep up. The possibility of eating free samples could not derail me from the large walk-in cold section that waited behind thick slats of clear plastic. Then I stopped.

"What is it?" Kerri asked.

I was having second thoughts. Did being in this wholesale big-box store make sense? Was shopping here true to the spirit of our project? If we bought food here, would we have to factor in the cost of the membership? How would we do that? By cost per day, or by dividing our annual membership dues by the number of visits? I realized that we could decide later.

"Let's just see what they have," I said.

Kerri got her phone and, using the calculator, figured out what we could afford. Before long there was a ten-pound bag of carrots in the cart. Then a five-pound bag of broccoli. Then we found the lettuce: six hearts of romaine for $2.39. It was too good to be true. It seemed impossible to buy produce at the traditional grocery store, given our extreme budget, and at the dollar store we were limited to onions and garlic. Today was different—we could actually afford to buy produce here. The idea of a salad resonated in my imagination as the questions over membership fees echoed in my psyche, but the power of fresh produce was too strong. Kerri placed the lettuce in the cart. Feeling inspired, we moved out of the cold section and on to the bags of apples and oranges, but they were still too expensive.

Having drunk nothing but water over the last two weeks, I wondered if we could manage a powdered drink mix. Heading up and down the aisles, we looked at all the food we couldn't afford, until finally we found it: Tang. The canister had images of orange slices emblazoned across the front, accented by an info-graphic proclaiming that this newly improved beverage contained "fruitrition." We tossed the item into our sparsely inhabited cart and made for the checkout stand. I was ecstatic. We would have salad with dinner that night, and orange drink with our oatmeal in the morning. Feeling enthused on the drive home, I made a spontaneous stop at a large fruit stand on the side of the road. The enormous sign out front advertised fresh local strawberries. Kerri gave me a funny look.

"We won't be able to afford anything here."

Smiling, I grabbed my wallet. "I'm just going to take a look."

The pyramids of locally grown fruits and vegetables were overwhelming, and the prices were surprisingly manageable even for modest budgets. However, as I looked around, I found little that we could afford. I made a mental note to remember this place for when the project was over. Then I saw them: oranges, a five-pound bag for five dollars. I counted the number in the bag; they were eighteen cents each. I realized that we could each have half an orange in our lunches. Our daily totals had been well below a dollar for the last few days, and I figured that we could manage this. Worries of getting sick would be a thing of the past. The baseball-sized blasts of citrus would save us. I pulled out a five-spot and handed it to the guy behind the makeshift counter. Walking back to the car, I held up the bag in victory. Kerri was shaking her head in disbelief. Once in the car, I explained the cost per orange, and she seemed just as pleased. I had no idea that today's thrifty victories would lead to a nickel-sized blunder the next day.

By our third week of eating on a dollar a day, it was clear that we had underestimated the power of food as a driving force in our lives. We knew we were hungry, but in addition our experiment had left us emotionally brittle, physically drained, and decidedly desperate for a more diverse diet. The next day it happened: I spent too much. It wasn't just the addition of Tang to our morning routine that put my daily total over a dollar. We also made polenta for dinner, and for the first time, we had a small salad with dressing as well. The dressing alone was eighteen cents a tablespoon, not a wise decision. Too many new things at once sent me over the top. Kerri's self-denial of a spot of peanut butter that morning was what enabled her to narrowly escape the extra five cents. I felt bad at first, but I learned my lesson. It wouldn't happen again.

It got me thinking, though: How was it that one tablespoon of salad dressing was the same price as an orange? And why was I willing to spend nearly 20 percent of my daily food budget on a salad topping, while questioning the possibility of eating a whole orange with my lunch? In a food system where large companies look to maximize profits at every turn, it makes sense that processed foods have a higher markup than fresh fruits and vegetables. And once one stops to think about where most of the money in the food system is made, it becomes clear why processed foods are the primary focus. This is where nearly all advertising dollars are spent, and where most food research and development takes place. There isn't very much "processing" to an orange. Someone planted it, grew it, picked it, and shipped it, in some cases adding it to a bag of other oranges for a bulk purchase. But with the salad dressing, several ingredients are required, meaning that there are more people and machines involved in the process. But what really matters is that no longer am I simply buying oil mixed with herbs and spices; there has been "value added" to these raw ingredients.

The fact that companies can "add value" to raw materials is what enables them to mark up these foods and sell them for the prices that they do. The food company is offering you a service. When you buy bread, you are not just buying flour, water, salt, and sugar (which is what most breads are made of)—you are buying something altogether different, and the differences lie in what value has been added. So instead of just selling one kind of bread, you are given a variety of choices: white, wheat, whole wheat, honey wheat, whole grain, heart-healthy, vitamin-enriched, made with prune juice for help with "digestion," etc. Anyone who has spent time in the bread aisle of a modern grocery store knows that the number of possible bread products and their advertised differences are nothing short of a dizzying array that would confound any sensible person. Yet consumers today have become more than just immune to this—we expect it.

In most cases, the ingredients list is far longer than most shoppers have time to read, and the ingredients that have been added are written in a scientific jargon that one needs a degree, or access to the Internet, to understand. All added ingredients have a purpose and add some type of "value" to the product. Sometimes a substitute is used to make the end product cheaper, to maintain its freshness, to reduce fat content, to provide more nutrients, to reduce calories, and so on.

It's harder to do the same thing with produce, as there isn't much value that can be added to something like lettuce. No matter what, it is just lettuce. A store can offer different varieties of leafy greens, but the options pale in comparison to the eereal aisle, or any other aisle, for that matter. Of course, some of the value added to our foods have hidden costs that we don't realize: low wages for workers, pollution from the creation and production of the product, animal cruelty, and of course the possible negative health impacts from eating too many of these types of foods.

In addition to the variety of products made possible by adding value, there are other ways for companies to add value as well, but the most common is the convenience factor. We have grown accustomed to purchasing foods that take little time or skill to prepare and require very little cleanup. Frozen dinners, which struggled to catch on until people could afford to have freezers in their homes, can be stored indefinitely, popped in the microwave, eaten in front of the television, and easily disposed of afterward. Canned soup is another example. Processed foods like these have the added value of saving people time. These types of foods found their footing in the fifties, when women were still doing most of the cooking, and several companies, and even the president of Campbell's Soup, claimed that these products were popular because they were saving women time, saving them from the drudgery of "slaving in the kitchen." Even in 1969, after married women had started to become a regular part of the workforce, the chairman of the board of the Corn Products Company said he believed that processed foods, made for the sake of convenience, were the cause of a "social revolution." He believed that the food industry had given women the "gift of time" and that this could allow them to "reinvest in bridge, canasta, garden club, and other perhaps soul-satisfying pursuits." Looking back, it is funny to think that of all things to cite as contributors to the struggle for women's equality, some men in the food industry believed that products like canned ravioli played a vital role.

But even if the food companies overestimated their role in the women's liberation movement, their innovations did revolutionize the amount of time people spent at home preparing food. We were learning this firsthand. Having been accustomed to picking up a loaf of bread at the store, or dropping a couple cans of refried beans into the cart, we were experiencing this loss of convenience on a daily basis. In the 1930s, it took people about two and a half hours in the kitchen each day to prepare food; in 2010, we spend on average roughly eight minutes.

On our first night, I had rolled out tortillas by hand—tortillas which would have cost me just a couple dollars at the grocery store. On the weekends, I watched Kerri prepare several different types of meals to eat during the week. While we could have spent that time at the beach instead, that would have meant that we would spend most of our evenings working in the kitchen after getting home from working all day. Plus, certain foods had to be planned for in advance. Dried beans, for instance, had to be soaked overnight.

Beyond saving money, the most noticeable benefit was that, for the first time in our entire lives, we knew exactly what we were eating. It was not the best food we had ever eaten, but it wasn't bad, and we felt a certain level of pride in knowing what we were putting into our bodies. We also learned that there is little reason to buy things like bread, tortillas, boxed Spanish rice, and refried beans. We now knew how to make these things, and they were far cheaper when made at home. What was even better was that they didn't take all that much know-how or energy to prepare.

For most of that third week, things stayed pretty routine. The added benefit of a small salad with dinner each night was wonderful. While the chopped-up hearts of romaine lettuce didn't add much to our daily calorie count, they did act as a sort of psychological lubricant to keep us feeling confident as the days passed by. I had already lost nine pounds by this point, and although I was still a few pounds above my ideal body weight, I could feel other signs of physical distress. My body ached to get more active. I thought about going to the gym, but the fact that I felt light-headed if I stood up too quickly reminded me that I simply did not have the calories to burn. I needed every ounce of energy just to make it through the day. Kerri felt similarly. She had stopped riding her bike to school, and her e-mails to me throughout the day were like mirror signals in a maximum-security prison. She, too, was thinking about food nonstop. It didn't help that my students wanted an update each morning on how things were going, and eventually I just started referring them to the blog so that I could try to think about something besides eating.

By the third Friday, we needed a change. For three weeks we had been going nonstop. Long workdays, and weekends spent preparing foods and cleaning the house, left little time for us to relax together. We decided to go to the movies. In general, Kerri and I don't spend very much money entertaining ourselves. For the most part, we spend our free time reading, watching a movie at home, or taking the dogs to the park. Kerri likes to crochet, and I like to think up new things to do, like trying to eat on a dollar a day. But that night we would eat our small bowl of broccoli-potato soup with a side salad and then head out for a night on the town.

While waiting in line under the lights outside the theater, we noticed that the price of admission seemed different tonight. The price was always nine dollars per person, and while we usually groan at the cost of tickets, this time it seemed like downright robbery. Nine dollars was nine days' worth of food for each of us. The cost for two hours of entertainment for us both (eighteen dollars) was nearly equivalent to how much we each had spent on food individually for the last three weeks (twenty-one dollars apiece—seven dollars per week, per person).

As the line inched forward, we thought of all the other ways that people spend their income. If one used the amount of purchasable food as the measure of its value, most things seemed monstrously overpriced. The designer coffee the woman in front of us sipped was three days' worth of food. The *New York Times* under the arm of her date was another few day's worth of sustenance. Put in these terms, my new phone was equal to nearly an entire year's worth of food. Sure, it could use GPS to give me my location, and I could check my e-mail at any moment, but did I really need my phone to tell me that I was at the movie theater in Del Mar? While this comparison might not have been entirely fair, it gave us a lot to consider. The stark contrast between the privileges afforded to us and the dire situations of those living in the developing world was troubling. While we hadn't started this project with any type of political agenda, the political implications that surfaced as a result of our experiences were becoming apparent.

Kerri and I often talked with others about those who have no choice but to live on a dollar a day. We listened to people as they told us that third-world poverty and eating on a dollar a day in the United States were not comparable; we wondered what they really meant, and how they knew this. Our questions about poverty were growing; questions about how a person could live on a dollar a day turned to questions about purchasing-power parity. Reflecting on the cost of canned tomatoes pushed me to wonder about the plight of the workers who harvested them. Our little project to see if we could eat for less was producing questions that seemed to unravel our understanding about how the world worked. Food seemed to be at the center of everything, and pulling at one strand forced us to consider things that we hadn't anticipated thinking about.

Is it true that 26,000 children die from poverty every day? How many people entered the twenty-first century without the ability to read or sign their names? How many people live without electricity? Is it true that the wealthiest country on Earth has the widest gap between rich and poor? Being at the movies, a night that was supposed to be a break from all of these thoughts, a time to relax and appreciate being together, had turned into a meditation on issues related to poverty. Of course, the most obvious realization was that if we were actually in a situation where we couldn't afford to eat more than a dollar's worth of food, we wouldn't be at the movies. We took our tickets from the teenage girl behind the glass and I smiled at Kerri; my student discount had saved us a dollar, a whole day's worth of food.

Once we stepped inside the theater, we watched as people lined up for snacks, the cost of which made them but a distant dream for us. The smell of movie theater popcorn has got to be one of the best food aromas on the planet, but tonight we wouldn't be able to take part in this calorie-laden custom. My tiny dinner had left room in my stomach, and I longed for a box of Sour Patch Kids and a cherry cola to pacify me as the previews started. The sounds of patrons ripping into their candy bars and the soft swishing of ice in their gigantic cups of soda were nearly unbearable.

This ritual of snacking on sweets while entering into the fantasy of film is a powerful combination. Doctors often tell parents not to let their children sit in front of the television with a bowl of chips or any other snacks, as it encourages mindless eating and in turn plays a role in the development of bad eating habits and overweight kids. Apparently, my parents didn't get the memo. I was a chubby kid in elementary school, and throughout high school some of my baby fat still clung to my face. I spent most of my youth playing baseball and running around outside; I rode my bike to school and I even played ice hockey as a teenager, but it was never enough to burn off the calories from what I ate.

My parents told me to eat everything on my plate, whether I liked it or not. Sitting at the dinner table, my father used to force me to eat Brussels sprouts, and the little green balls seemed to weigh fifty pounds as I lifted each one from my plate. I would save my milk so that I could flood my mouth to wash them down. Even today, Brussels sprouts seem enormous, and I have yet to eat one as an adult. I would have rather chowed down on Kraft mac and cheese and washed away the delicious residue with a 7UP, or ordered a pizza from Pizza Hut.

By the time I turned thirteen, that had become more common. My parents had divorced a year earlier, and family dinners were rare. My mother worked long hours and took classes at night, so convenience foods became the norm. I remember the nights when she would make pork chops and applesauce or meat loaf, but more frequent were the evenings of Campbell's bean with bacon soup, or hot dogs with the little cheese bits inside. Fresh fruits and vegetables didn't play even a supporting role. My sister and I were only at my dad's house, where we ate a lot of pizza and had big breakfasts at a place called Paradise Grill, every other weekend.

At school, the food was no better. For lunch I would buy one of the large chocolate chip cookies and a soda. After school, I ate fast food with my friends. When my best friend got his license, it meant late nights at the Taco Bell drive-through, which was open twenty-four hours, and at the McDonald's just up the street for twenty-nine-cent-cheeseburger night. Every Wednesday we would order ten burgers each and a whole tray of fries and eat until we couldn't move. We knew it wasn't the best food choice, but we had little idea how unhealthy it really was. My health teacher in high school was a large man who sat at the front of the class with a Super Big Gulp in one hand and one of those large microwave burritos in the other. He looked like a sweaty bear and did nothing to model what he was supposed to be teaching us (and this was at one of *Newsweek*'s "100 Best High Schools" in the nation). The result of having been raised on these food options is that I have struggled with my weight for most of my life. I have never been obese, but I have been consistently ten to twenty pounds overweight. I grew up with the habit of eating everything in front of me, most of which happened to be energy-dense foods laden with fat and coated with sugar. Physical activity was more an occasional thing than a way of life.

As an adult, I still fall victim to these foods every now and then, and while I have gotten better about exercising, if I am not diligent, my waistline will grow. Part of this is because I love sweets. Cookies, cupcakes, brownies, candy, and anything with chocolate are all temptations that I struggle to resist. Kerri's mom knows this about me and indulges the habit when we visit them during the holidays. I can always count on a box of Cap'n Crunch on top of her fridge, and Double Stuf Oreos on the counter. As if loading up on sugar in the morning wasn't bad enough, every time I walk through the kitchen, a cookie seems to land in my mouth, sometimes two.

During this experiment, we couldn't afford such high-calorie treats. However, the batch of peanut butter cookies I baked as a peace offering for Kerri the week before, and the nightly tablespoons of peanut butter sweetened with high-fructose corn syrup, were enough to keep me from having sugar withdrawals. As an adult, I take full responsibility for my dietary choices, but I also recognize that my formative years were shaped by the strategies of food marketing experts, omnipresent fast food, and my parents' need for cheap and easy mealtime solutions. For the first time, I was doing my best to unlearn what I knew about eating, and I was working to unpack more than twenty years of food baggage.

By the time the weekend had started, Kerri was back to work getting our meals ready for the week. I cleaned around the house while she soaked beans, made soup, baked bread, and prepared wheat gluten cutlets for dinner. To the independent observer, it would have seemed that she had been doing this her entire life, as Kerri's ability to multitask in the kitchen was beyond inspiring. Although she moved gracefully around the kitchen, I could tell that she was veering toward total exhaustion. I started to feel guilty for convincing her to go through with this. It had been my idea, and now I could see Kerri working hard in the kitchen and nearing the brink of burnout. I, too, was feeling less energetic, but overall I had grown accustomed to eating smaller-sized portions. I felt liberated from packaged and highly processed foods, and I was proud that we had actually made it that far. In addition, while I knew that it was unhealthy for me to lose so much weight so quickly, I was secretly delighted that I might end this experiment looking better than when we started.

A Friend for Dinner

Kerri

By Tuesday of our last week, I felt miserable. All I wanted to do was collapse on the couch. I have never been one to call in sick. When I was younger, this was because I couldn't afford a day off, but as a teacher, it's a pain to call in. In past jobs, calling in sick wasn't a big deal. Someone higher up called another employee in to work while I went back to bed. I didn't have to think about anything. In teaching, it's not that easy. As a group, most teachers don't call in sick unless we are truly miserable. I am sure it isn't that we are sick less frequently than people in other professions, but some days it feels like it takes less effort to come in sick than to make lesson plans for a substitute and make sure all materials are easy to access. However, it really is surprising that teachers are not sick more often. Imagine a hundred people coming through your workspace in a single day— coming in sick themselves, touching doorknobs, sneezing on desks, and coughing. A classroom is one big germ party.

On Monday I started to feel sick, and on Tuesday, work was miserable. I love my students, but during the course of a single day, I see more than one hundred of them, and they all need something. It can be overwhelming when I'm feeling fine, but when I'm ill, it's difficult to cope with. I often tell my students that I am happy to answer their questions as long as they don't swarm me; otherwise, after class they will surround my desk. I finished off the day on Tuesday, but I needed to stay late because I had made a decision. I would call in sick the next day. I needed extra time that evening to prepare for the sub.

I only had a sore throat and a headache, so I probably could have gone to school the next day and survived, but I didn't want to put any more strain on my body than I already had. I was running out of energy and I felt exhausted. If I kept pushing forward, I might really get sick. With only one week to go, I wanted to make sure we survived without any major illnesses. That does not change the fact that whenever I miss a day, I feel guilty, as if I am somehow letting my students down. They probably don't feel that way, but I worry about it. When I'm not in the classroom, it's hard to rest because I'm concerned about what's going on in my absence. Are they doing what they need to be doing? Is the sub following my lesson plans? But, in the end, sick days are supposed to be used when I need them, and I should be taking that time to recover instead of spreading my germs around.

I have an allotted number of sick days every year, so I wouldn't be losing any pay for taking a day to recover. In my previous jobs, a loss of a day meant a loss of pay, and that is a reality for many people. They are then forced to make a choice that has several repercussions: going to work sick and not taking the time to get over the illness; risking making a small problem worse; spreading the infection to coworkers and customers. On the other hand, calling in sick might mean a loss of wages for one or more days; problems paying bills or being able to pay for a doctor's visit; and, in the worst cases, even losing the job.

It was my turn to post on our blog that night, and I wrote about my ailments. It was important to let our readers know how we were faring, but if there was any way we could have blocked our parents from reading our blogs that last week, I am sure that we would have. I usually talk to my parents a couple of times a week, and both of them were concerned with our health. Whenever I spoke with my dad, one of his first questions was how were we feeling. He claimed that every time I spoke to him, I sounded tired or worn down.

"How's everything going?"

"Fine, Dad. I just had a long day."

"Oh, is that it? I thought you sounded a little tired. I can hear it in your voice. How much longer until you guys are finished?"

"A couple more days, don't worry. I'm fine, really. How's Mom?"

I tried to find a way to allay his fears as fast as I could and move on to other issues. Christopher's mom was worse. Her concern became pervasive by the fourth week. Lynda is also a teacher, and as part of a nutrition unit that she was teaching, which happened to correspond with our project, her fifth-grade class was following our adventures. It seemed that her class was starting to be concerned about us, so she kept calling to pass that on. Their fears heightened her own, and rarely a day went by that we didn't hear from her. Lynda meant well, and we knew she was just worried, but on more than one occasion she left us a long message on our answering machine, telling us it was time to stop the dollar project. She didn't want us to continue, even though we only had a few days left. Each message she left was longer and sterner than the last. "Okay, you two, this has gone on long enough and you could get really sick. You need to stop this now. I'm serious." It got to the point that when she called, we let the phone ring and turned the volume down while she left a message.

This is not to say that there was no validity to the concerns of our loved ones. I often tell my students that they need to eat breakfast and a healthy lunch in order to perform well. Trying to focus on an empty stomach severely impacts learning. Despite such admonishments to my students, however, we had ignored our own warnings and plunged into a monthlong "do as I say, not as I do" experiment. We learned quickly that hunger is time-consuming. When you're hungry, it's easier to pay attention to your growling gut than to whatever may be going on in class. Any full day of school or work is exhausting, even if you have plenty to eat. When you're missing the calories or nutrients needed to make it through the day, the tasks ahead are even more daunting. If students are coming to school hungry, they are probably not getting the same thing out of the school day that a well-fed classmate is.

In addition to the impact on our work lives, the lack of variety caused unexpected effects. Eating a diet low in diversity posed problems for our taste buds, but also, more importantly, to our health. For the first day of our project we took vitamin supplements, but then we realized that purchasing vitamins was not within our daily budget. We talked about calculating the cost, but we didn't want to sacrifice the extra few cents' worth of food that supplementing our diet might have taken away from us. We were more concerned about full bellies than checking whether or not we met the recommended daily allowance (RDA) of nutrients every day. Whether or not this was nutritionally the right choice, we weren't sure. However, it seemed more important to eat enough than to make sure we met the RDA.

Advertisements push for people to consume vitamin-enriched foods, rather than a wide enough variety of foods so that most nutrients can be acquired naturally. There is an abundance of enriched foods in grocery stores, and some of the nutrients that the items are enriched with are the same ones that were lost in the refining or processing of it. "Enriched" on a food label indicates that the nutrients were added back to the same level that was lost in the processing. "Fortified" means that the nutrients were added at a level higher than what the food originally contained. It is unclear what the benefits are of adding nutrients to processed foods, as opposed to eating a variety of foods with naturally occurring benefits. And while there are many foods that are enriched, they tend to be the ones that are less healthful to begin with. Walking down the cereal aisle of a grocery store, the message is clear. The boxes are labeled with "9 essential nutrients," or "Now with calcium," which can be misleading to consumers and translated into "healthy." However, I strongly believe that eating a neon-colored artificially flavored fruit cereal will not have the same health benefits of a whole grain cereal with fresh fruit, even if the cereal is "enriched."

The whole idea of enriching foods came around after World War I. Soldiers had been rejected from the military due to poor health, and it was understood that strong Americans would make a stronger America. Other attempts to get people to consume the RDA for nutrients didn't include helping them to diversify their diet or to make nutritious food less expensive, but instead enriching the foods people already ate with nutrients. This enriching of foods continues today, when even more foods are processed and in need of nutrients. Ambiguity and lack of government regulation give companies the upper hand in labeling products with health claims, even when such health claims may be misleading.

We had weren't eating anything neon-colored, and what we ate wasn't necessarily bad for us. Our issues came more from the fact that our dollar-a-day portions were too small for us to get the calories we needed to function, and our limited repertoire of dishes partnered with the meager amount of fruits and vegetables we could afford didn't supply a wide range of nutrients. While we longed for something different, we still savored what little we had. It was hard to imagine eating less than we were, but on one night that week, we did.

We had promised a friend of ours, my coworker Dave, that we would have him over for dinner at some point during our project. Due to other commitments on both sides, the meal had been pushed back to this last week. In addition to teaching, Dave is also a freelance writer for a few local publications, and he wanted to write an article about what we were doing. We had known since the start of our project that Dave would be coming over for dinner one night, and on our twenty-fifth day, a Thursday, we finally were able to make it happen.

With the exception of a trip to the movies and our outing to a lecture at a university, during the dollar project Christopher and I had spent little time, outside of work, with other people. We tend to be homebodies, but we do occasionally make an effort to get out and see people. However, in the past month, our routine had turned into a never-ending cycle of eat, work, prepare food, eat, blog, bed. It was getting to be monotonous. We had never paid attention to how much of our social time revolved around food.

The social nature of eating left us feeling secluded. Several times during that month, I was invited to meet friends for lunch or coffee, and each time I declined. I could have gone and not ordered anything, but it would have been torturous to sit and smell the food and watch people enjoying tasty treats that I couldn't have, even though they were right in front of me. Food is more than what we need to keep our bodies running. Food helps us interact socially; it is part of what we do to entertain. When I have people over, I like to try new recipes with ingredients that we don't typically have at home. I usually have some type of appetizer and dessert, which we don't do every night when it's just the two of us. I have a tendency to overdo it for guests and special occasions, often making enough food to feed twice as many as we have invited. Like most people, I want to make sure that my guests go home full and happy.

Our dinner with Dave was different. He was coming over to see how things were going and to sample what we had been eating. While I did want to make sure he enjoyed his meal, I was also well aware of the fact that Christopher and I would each have a little less that day, as our rule stated that guests must eat from our share. We decided on this rule because we knew that when money is tight, more does not magically appear just because there's an extra mouth to feed. I also knew that Dave would most likely go home and eat something more. Still, while serving dinner, we made sure that each of us received an equal portion.

As we sat down to eat, I anxiously awaited Dave's response to our menu. Although beans, rice, homemade tortillas, and potatoes were a dish that we were now overly familiar with, our version was going to be new to our guest. I wondered what was going through his mind as he lifted the little burrito to his mouth. As he chewed, I could see the surprise on his face. He hadn't expected it to taste good.

All of the food we ate tasted good, except for one bean soup that I'd made. Christopher would disagree, but he'll eat almost anything. We never had to eat things that tasted horrible. It was more that some of the dishes were a bit bland, our portions were much smaller than we were used to—and again, the lack of variety. By the time we had Dave over for dinner, it was the second time that week that we had eaten that meal, and we would have it at least one more time before the week was over. The lack of variety not only bored our taste buds, but also left us wanting more.

I searched for a way to make that "more" seem tangible. For this entire month, I was constantly thinking about food: how little I had eaten, what I would be eating next, and whether or not it would fill me up. By this time, I was well into "window shopping." Under the pretext of looking for new recipes that called for few ingredients, I frequently got out several of my cookbooks and flipped through the pages. I dreamed of what I would eat when we were done and imagined the shopping trips where I could put anything I wanted into the cart. In some of the cookbooks were sticky notes that tagged our favorites, and others that I wanted to try. After dinner I sometimes tormented Christopher by saying, "You know what sounds good right now?"

Usually I only intended to tell him one thing that I wanted, but it wouldn't take long for my "want" list to spiral out of control. "I'd like a salad" turned into "with a side of mashed potatoes and something chocolate, followed by baked tofu and salsa." At that point I fell into listing every food I had ever enjoyed in my lifetime. There is no questioning who the weak link was, but more often than not, Christopher jumped in with one or two dream meals of his own. However, these dreams had to be put on hold; my cookbooks needed to tide me over for a few more days. The countdown to the end had started.

As he only ate one meal with us, for Dave, the lack of variety wasn't an issue. He said, "This is actually good," as he worked on his second burrito. He was right; it was good. We offered him a splash of Tang to wash it down. He was hesitant; he didn't want to take too much and leave us hungry, but his curiosity got the best of him and he tried it. He said it was just like he remembered from childhood. As we ate, we talked about our project and how we had been doing.

When we calculated our cost that evening, we were pleased to see that we could afford to each have a cookie. Dave mentioned that he was impressed by the portion sizes we were able to feed him. He had almost stopped to eat something before he came over, but he said he was glad he didn't. Of course, the next day I asked him if he had eaten when he got home. He said, "Not right away," but he did have a snack later that evening.

We had a few days left before we could rejoin the world of late-night snacking. I felt as if I had a better understanding of why weight-loss diets fail so often. My mind was consumed by all of the items I was deprived of. My situation was artificial; I could have quit anytime, and the foods I wanted were in reach. If I wanted them, I could have had them. I was tempted. I wanted something new; a new flavor. Despite the fact that we were almost done, we cracked, but just a little. Our rules stated that we would only have our packaged ramen noodles if there was no other way to stay under budget. On our last Saturday, we were short on time and needed something fast to eat for lunch. By this point, we were looking for an excuse to eat the ramen. I offered it as a suggestion, sure that Christopher would shoot it down, but he agreed without any prodding. When I confessed that it actually sounded *good* to me, I didn't expect him to concur, but he did.

We rationalized that there wasn't time to make something else, but in reality, we probably could have managed. The truth was that we were excited. Tearing open the blue packaging and seeing the crispy noodles made me happy. My brain took a quick trip down memory lane to elementary school when I had just learned of the miracles of ramen. At that time, it wasn't uncommon for kids in my school to crunch up a package of uncooked noodles, sprinkle the flavor package on it, and eat it as a snack. I was sure that I was guilty of this at some point in time. I also thought back to all the jokes about starving college students eating only ramen noodles to survive, and how proud I was that I made it through my first year without ever buying a package; maybe working at a grocery store gave me other options. Now here I was at twenty-nine years old, waiting for the water to boil so I could let my noodles cook for the requisite two minutes before I could sprinkle in the salty, MSG-laden contents of the little silver packet.

I never thought I would be so thrilled by such a meal, but I was almost giddy with excitement after my first bite. The warm, salty broth was just what I needed, and the noodles were such a wonder-fully different texture and taste from the white rice and potatoes that had been so prevalent in our diet. However, as is typical of ra-men, it sounded like a good plan, and the first several bites were great, but as we finished our bowls, sure to get every last slurp of the broth, it no longer seemed like a great idea. My stomach was already saying, "Why did you do that?" I worried about what toll it would take on Christopher, who had been battling stomach issues for the past twenty-four hours. But I didn't regret it. It was the new flavor I needed. Now I'd had it, and I was over it.

My food daydreams continued, though. One of my favorite guilty pleasures is eating a fluffy, chocolate-covered donut. When I was little, my dad used to take my sisters and me to get donuts on Sunday mornings before church, and my favorite is forever the chocolate bar. One problem I run into is that there are very few bakeries that make vegan donuts. The closest one I know of is in Las Vegas, which hap-pens to be over five hours away if traffic is clear. Fortunately, our friends Spencer and Stacy have family in Las Vegas, and every time they go, they bring a box back to us. They called us on Sunday and asked us if we wanted them to bring some. They knew we were ap-proaching the end of our project, and they could bring them by on Monday—but we wouldn't be able to eat them until Wednesday.

Christopher passed the decision off to me, but I felt the answer was obvious. I wanted them. It would be difficult to have them sit on our counter and not eat them, but we had made it twenty-eight days—two more would be a breeze. When they arrived, I had Christopher put the box in the cupboard above our refrigerator: out of sight, out of mind. But that wasn't really the case. I was acutely aware of the pink box of wonder that lingered just beyond the reach of my fingertips. Anytime I walked into the kitchen I would inhale deeply, as if I could actually taste them if only I could get enough of their scent.

But these donuts spurred another conversation in our house. How would we eat after this project? We knew that we were begin-ning to look at food differently, and now we needed to discuss how this would impact the way we shopped and lived. While our wallets, and not our health, were the initial focus, we had learned that healthy foods were something we valued, our sweet tooth notwith-standing. We liked starting from whole foods to make our meals, but we wanted variety, and we craved fruits and vegetables. One of our observations was that we would need to be willing to spend more time planning and preparing our meals if we wanted to avoid the boxed and canned convenience foods from before. Not to say that we planned never to eat anything that might be bad for us, or that we had only eaten "healthy" foods before this, but we were now looking for a more healthful diet. Perhaps not the first day. After all, there were perfectly good three-day-old donuts to consider.

Despite the fact that the week before I would have said I thought it would never end, on our last day I couldn't believe that our month had gone by so quickly. Still, I had no desire to continue. While I lost half as much weight as Christopher had, for my size it still felt like too much. During my free period at school, I used a pair of scissors to poke a new hole in my belt. I would be visiting my parents the next week, and I knew they would tell me that I was too skinny.

On the last day, I headed to the grocery store after work to get some food for our lunches the next day. Christopher had called me with two requests: Tofurkey slices and strawberries. This would be the first time I had been to a grocery store, other than a bulk store, in over thirty days. I wasn't prepared for it. It had been so long since I had walked under that much fluorescence; when I walked in, the lights felt like an assault on my vision. But that wasn't the hardest part. I knew we only needed those two items, but I grabbed a basket and wandered. The vibrant reds, greens, and oranges of the produce section were juxtaposed against the different variations of white, beige, and brown that had graced my plate for a month. I was overwhelmed. I found strawberries on sale, and then worked my way back toward the refrigerated section. I considered going back to the front of the store to get a cart. I wanted to load up and gain the security that comes from having a full cabinet and knowing that food is there if I need it.

Several times I put crackers or chips or other snack-type food in my basket, only to take it out when I realized I didn't really need it. But I kept wandering. Twice I called Christopher to have him talk me out of things. I knew that with the donuts, we didn't need more sugar in our house, but didn't he think that soy ice cream sounded good? Did he want chips and salsa as a snack tomorrow? There was a game show that used to be on when I was in high school, and at one point in the game, the customers had a limited amount of time to run through the store and get as many items as they could into their cart. I think the object was to make the checkout total as high as possible. That day, I wanted to run through the store and, with grand sweeping motions, knock everything I could reach into my cart. I wanted to fill my car with full grocery bags so that I could replenish my Mother Hubbard cupboards. But I didn't. I was reasonable, mostly. I cruised the aisles for at least twenty minutes, but in the end, I went home with my two items.

That night, we had our last meal for under a dollar. With the dishes done and the blog posted, we went to bed early. The next day would be a whole new start for us. We would be reintroduced into the world of food. I could have coffee, and I wouldn't be eating oatmeal, not for a long, long time. We were filled with so much anticipation that it was almost like the night before Christmas—but instead of sugar plums, I had visions of chocolate bar donuts dancing in my head.

The Aftermath

Christopher

Like any other day, I opened my eyes to the darkness of morning and rolled out of bed to get ready for work, but today was different from those that had come before it. Our month of eating on a dollar a day had ended. I should have felt more excited, but like birthdays and other big celebrations, often the anticipation of a particular moment is greater than its arrival. The vegan donuts that our friends Spencer and Stacy brought back from Ronald's Donuts in Las Vegas were waiting patiently in their big pink box. Most people would probably see the eating of a three-day-old donut as disgusting; some would call the excitement over said baked goods patently absurd. But as a confessed sugar addict who had forgone a necessity like chocolate for a month, this custard-filled chocolate bar donut was nothing short of a climax for the taste buds. The feeling was probably similar to what addicts feel once they finally get a fix: pure ecstasy, with a recognition of how good it feels to be bad once again—a victory for our darker natures.

Our doctor had recommended that when this project was over, we make sure not to overdo it on our first day back. He cited those people imprisoned in death camps during World War II who had died shortly after being released because they overworked their starved bodies by eating too much. They literally ate themselves to death. Our experience was nothing in comparison, but we appreciated the advice and would not make the same mistake. Surely a donut was acceptable.

That the treat had lost some of its doughy nature was easily forgotten as my teeth found the smooth vanilla custard, and my tongue lapped up the excess chocolate frosting. After the first few bites, the foreplay was over and I got down to the business of militant chewing, only to be interrupted by momentary breaks to wash down the bites. Today there would be no Tang. The sugar from my breakfast dessert floated down my throat on a current of freshly squeezed juice from some of our leftover oranges. For a moment I rationalized that the nectar of this fresh fruit made up for what I was about to do next.

Kerri emerged from the bathroom with a towel wrapped around her head, and I smiled as I popped open the lid of the pink box to survey my options. I would be good. I would not reach for the spectacular swirls of the cinnamon roll; that would be too much. The jelly-filled dusted with powdered sugar would have been an elegant option, but the raspberry gel seemed a touch extravagant. I settled on another chocolate bar, this one unfilled—an obvious and reasonable choice. The oatmeal that had occupied a place in our daily morning ritual had officially become a thing of the past, a tradition easily discarded for a new era in eating. I would once again revel in the variety of the American food system. I could go back to having fruit smoothies, or cereal with fresh fruit before work, and French toast with soy sausage on the weekends.

I watched Kerri as she delicately enjoyed her own sweet relief. The bliss of our morning breakfast seemed to settle our souls. We had made it through a month of frugal dining that left us exhausted, and we were overjoyed to get back to life as usual. No more weighing, calculating, and rationing out meager portions. No more feelings of desperation or frustration at the thought of cooking something that would leave us only mildly satisfied. No more worries about getting the proper amounts of nutrients. No more fighting over cookies. I said good-bye to Kerri and left for work with a new sense of satisfaction. We had made it; we had survived for one month eating on a dollar each a day.

I blasted the car stereo on the way to work, with the chorus of Minor Threat's "Stepping Stone" giving me an added air of accomplishment. The first thing my students asked when we started class was, "What did you have for breakfast?" However, as I recounted the joy of our morning treat, I could feel my stomach rising up in protest. I worried that my body was breaking down from sugar overload. I wondered if I had overdone it. Would I throw up? Would I have diarrhea? Were the donuts too old? Would I end up like those unfortunate folks who ate too much after years of forced starvation? Sweating and starting to feel painfully uncomfortable, I did what any teacher would do. I put on a smile and faked it. I ate on a dollar a day for a month; I could manage a couple of donuts. At break I rushed to the bathroom and, sure enough, my body quickly rejected the foreign food. I felt better immediately, and by lunch I had no inhibitions about launching into my soy turkey sandwich and organic strawberries. The rest of the afternoon was a breeze, and the thought of eating out made me light with excitement. What was once commonplace was now novelty. To think that I could go to a place where people would prepare me a fantastic meal, and that I wouldn't have to worry about the cost, seemed reserved for mere fantasy.

After work, Kerri and I accompanied my mother to Sipz, one of our favorite restaurants in town. This vegetarian Asian-fusion cafe boasts a lengthy menu, and flipping through the pages was like being in the office of a travel agent and looking at all the places worth visiting and having to pick just one. I know that most foodies sneer at any establishment that calls itself "fusion," but Sipz pulls it off with style. Even our staunchly omnivorous family members request it when we get together.

First we ordered some summer rolls and mock-barbecue chicken for appetizers. Then we put in our entrees: pad Thai for Kerri, and mock chicken curry with broccoli for me. Of course our meal would have been incomplete without beverages, so I requested a taro-root boba slushie (tastes like a vanilla milk shake) and Kerri had an iced tea. My mother, who was taking us out to celebrate the end of our project, was happy to see us finally eating a proper amount of calories, and I think she would have paid for just about anything that night if we could have eaten it. When our bowls came out, the servings were enormous. These mountains of food could not possibly fit into our newly shrunken stomachs. I thought about the obesity rate in our country, and one of the causes was sitting on the plate right in front of me. The size of portions we are served at most restaurants is far more than we actually need, especially since most people lead relatively sedentary lives. I thought back to my high school days of overeating at fast-food joints and reminded myself that I did not have to finish everything served to me.

With every bite came a new level of satisfaction, but I paid closer attention to my body than usual. Having learned my lesson earlier that day, and having relayed it to Kerri, we ate about half of our dinners and boxed up the remainders for lunch the next day. As much as we enjoyed our food, our bodies still struggled to adjust. I have overeaten before and felt the oversaturation of too much food throughout my body, but this was different. This was not a typical food coma. My level of energy that night dipped below zero as my body poured most of its resources into helping me cope with the abundance of food working its way through my system. I couldn't help but toss and turn as I lay in bed and tried to fall asleep.

Over the course of the next few days, our bodies adjusted to eating reasonably sized portions, but our way of looking at everything related to food was forever changed. We continued to plan our weekly meal schedule, shop around for the best deals, and eat mostly unprocessed foods that could be bought in bulk as raw materials. The most significant change in our shopping trips was that we were able to reintroduce fresh fruits and vegetables, which healed our nutrient-deficient bodies and helped us regain confidence in our level of health. We started exercising again, and no longer did I feel lightheaded at work.

Our students noticed a difference, too. By the time the project was over, some of Kerri's students finally knew about it, and upon discussion in class, one student remarked, "So that's why you were so cranky last month." Kerri was quite surprised. Since they had known about it all along, my students had different observations. Although they tried to hide it, I could hear the chatter in the background, and one student had the courage to look me in the eye and say, "You look too skinny, Mr. Greenslate." While I had been quite pleased about shedding some excess weight, she had a point. In just thirty days I had lost fourteen pounds, or close to half a pound every day, and without any exercise. I couldn't tighten my belt any further, and my pants hung loose around my waist. Kerri had only lost five pounds, and while I couldn't tell that she had lost any weight, she often put her arms around me and exclaimed that I was disappearing right in front of her.

In fact, this was one of the things that readers of our blog were most worried about. Readers often posted questions asking about our weight loss, and others gave us medical explanations about what was going on with our health as a result of the experiment. In addition to readers' questions about how we were holding up, and comments meant to inspire us, people kept donating their money to the Community Resource fund, as well. I had asked our readers at one point to help us break the thousand-dollar mark, which I thought was pretty ambitious, considering that we were complete strangers to most of them. While my father and a few other family members made donations, we were seeing people from all over the world giving amounts from as little as a buck to one reader who handed over two hundred dollars after returning home from an evening out with friends to find our blog. The reader was matching what she had spent on dinner that night.

For the rest of October, we were focused on teaching and on getting our lives back to normal. Yet the donations sitting in our online account, and the large buckets of raw ingredients taking up space in our kitchen, stood as reminders that our project had changed our lives forever. We soon started to understand that there was something more powerful here than we had originally anticipated when we planned our survivalist experiment. This project started as a way to learn, an "experiment in truth," as Gandhi would say. We knew that at the very least we would no longer see food or grocery shopping the same way, but we had not really considered how other people would perceive the project. We soon found out.

As November approached, we had received e-mails from literary agents in New York, and then a call from Tara Parker-Pope, a health writer at *The New York Times*. In speaking with Tara, we discussed the details of our experiment and other issues related to food and global poverty. The journalism teacher in me was doing my best both to learn from speaking with her and to keep my guard up. But then she said something that surprised me. With a casual tone she said, "I am going to make you famous." I grew silent and smiled at the audacity of her comment. I myself have been known to say a thing or two that makes people do a double take. I laughed at the idea. Soon enough, we were back to talking about our monthlong dollar diet, and she requested a follow-up interview with Kerri at some point in the near future.

About a week later, on the day that our country elected its first African American president, the article came out. It was titled "Money Is Tight, and Junk Food Beckons." In addition to talking about our project, she also cited a study done by the director of the Center for Public Health and Nutrition at the University of Washington published in *The Journal of the American Dietetic Association* about how the cost of healthful food had risen by 19.5 percent over the course of the two-year study, whereas the cost of junk foods had actually decreased. The article also included a link to our blog.

As soon as the article was out, our readership went from respectable to astronomical. All of a sudden there were tens of thousands of people from around the country talking about our project. The next day the article was reprinted in *The International Herald-Tribune*, the international version of the *Times*. Our readership continued to grow, this time to a global audience. Before long we were getting e-mail and comments from people in Egypt, the Czech Republic, Brazil, and a whole host of other countries. Their comments on our project were fascinating. We watched as people argued over some of the claims in the article about the cost of healthful food. We witnessed people unload their political and economic philosophies on one another. And of course, lots of people shared their stories from college— mostly about being "poor" and eating ramen noodles.

What was most fascinating, though, was the fact that thousands of people had read the same story, read our blog, and come to entirely different conclusions. All of a sudden we had simultaneously proven both that one *could* eat well on a dollar a day, and that one could not. Each reader had drawn a different conclusion from our project, and often they were in direct contradiction to one another. Of course, having actually been the ones who did the project, we knew that it was more complex than this. It was clear, though, from our experience that it was very difficult to find affordable fresh food. At the same time, we couldn't have afforded a lot of junk foods either. What made the most sense was to eat mostly beans and rice and homemade soups, and to eat small portions. When we were lucky enough to eat carrots and lettuce, it felt like just that: lucky.

After the initial frenzy over the piece, which had more reader comments than any other article in the *New York Times* health section for the next few weeks, we started getting messages from other media organizations. All of a sudden we were being contacted by *The Oprah Winfrey Show*, the Canadian Broadcast Corporation, and *Inside Edition*. It was both bizarre and exciting, and it was just the beginning. While on a trip with my students to the Fall National High School Journalism Convention in St. Louis that next week, we did a live television appearance on the *News Hour*, aired across Canada, and a week later we had a small crew from *Inside Edition* following us around the Smart and Final store where we had bought most of our bulk items. As we don't subscribe to cable television, we had never seen the show *Inside Edition* before, and in retrospect were incredibly naive to think that any part of the forty-five-minute interview we did about poverty would end up in the segment as part of the show. When it finally aired, we had to go over to our friend Krista's house to watch it, and as it came on, we laughed to see our experience sandwiched between the birthday bash for Britney Spears and a walrus that could play the saxophone. The best part of the whole experience was that after the show, we got to spend time with one of our good friends and eat a delicious meal with fresh salad greens picked from her backyard garden.

We thought for sure that our ninety-second stint on a celebrity news show was the extent of our newfound "fame," but we were wrong. The next day we received an e-mail from a producer at the nationally aired morning television news show *Fox & Friends*. As much as I don't care for their organization, I wasn't about to pass up on the opportunity to talk to such a large audience about the cost of eating well. Plus, the audience for *Fox & Friends* would be relatively different from that of *The New York Times*. For all my feelings about the quality of reporting at Fox News, I must give them credit for not only picking up on a relevant concern for Americans, but also for treating us well. Since the show broadcasts live from New York, the time difference between coasts meant that we would have to be up at three a.m. in order to be in a satellite studio for our time slot. By three thirty, there was a car and driver in front of our house, waiting to take us downtown for the interview. By the time we got back home, we had thousands more visitors who had seen the blog, and just as before, the responses varied widely in perspective. Feeling good about the whole experience, we went back to sleep in order to feel a little more rested for a daylong work meeting.

We had a surprising amount of energy at the meeting. About half-way through the day, one of our colleagues approached us and said, "Hey, I saw you guys on Yahoo.com just a little while ago." Stunned, we went to the nearest computer and logged in. Sure enough, we were on the front page, with a video clip of the interview. The clip stayed online for the next few days, and through the weekend, and as a result, traffic to our blog jumped once again, at times reaching over 200,000 hits a day. It was official: Our little blog about our silly little project had reached an exponential number of people. It was funny to think that at the beginning, Kerri would chastise me for mentioning the idea of our project to the checker at our natural foods store, and now there were millions of people who had heard about it, and several hundred thousand who were visiting our site directly.

It was at this point that we started to realize the scope of the conversation we had entered. Reader comments on our blog were coming from everyone from cash-strapped moms in Tennessee and Arizona who were trying to feed their children on a limited income to personal finance specialists on Wall Street who were trying to give their clients tips on how to stretch their dollar even further during the recession. There were health care professionals in Riverside, California, and nutritionists in Pittsburgh, Pennsylvania; Peace Corps workers in South America and gardenistas from Chicago; food bank workers from Kentucky and people struggling with celiac disease—all making their way to our blog to learn about what we did. Instantly our site had turned into a place where all kinds of people were discussing everything from how to get the best deals in the grocery store to how to start a windowsill garden. From helping the hungry in our country to those starving in the third world. From nutrition tips to cancer treatment, and from government food policy to the practices of large agribusiness. Everyone from foodies to Wal-Mart exclusives were stopping by, and every avenue of the food discussion was in play.

From here, we had the opportunity to watch it all unfold and to learn from all the people who took the time to add their voices to the conversation. When I looked to see where readers were coming from to visit our site, I learned that they were hearing about our project all over the blogosphere as well. From the Whole Foods website to the Kenneth Cole site, and from all kinds of blogger moms to Earthfirst!, people were tuning in and responding. Very soon the level of donations doubled, and we felt it was necessary to meet up with the Community Resource Center and hand over the funds that had been collecting from generous readers worldwide.

Upon calling the Community Resource Center, I mentioned who the donations were coming from, and having heard about the project in our local paper, *The San Diego Union-Tribune*, they were very pleased to hear from us. As it grew clear that the nation was headed for recession, donations to nonprofits had been falling quickly, and for organizations like the Community Resource Center that provide all kinds of services for families, including food assistance, demand was growing. While I was on the phone with the woman from the center, she asked if we would like to attend their invitation-only reception the night before their annual holiday basket program began. We agreed, figuring that we would do a check presentation and meet some of the people who helped run the program.

When the evening arrived, my mother accompanied us to the event, which was being held at the Del Mar Fairgrounds. We entered the facility where things were being prepared for the following day and stood there in awe at the sight of the volunteers who were putting together "food baskets," grocery bags filled with donated food items. A dozen tables were lined up end to end with nearly thirty volunteers, ranging in age from eight to eighty, packing and filling boxes with food for the following day's opening of the Holiday Basket Program.

During that weekend, over 1,200 families were given the chance to have a dignified "shopping experience" as they would make their way through the huge hallway and pick up items that would help them make it through the holidays. With the economic downturn, programs like this—run entirely by donations and thousands of volunteer hours—are a testament to the power of community. Participating in this moment was both instructive and inspiring. We left the reception amazed by what happens when people work together to get things done for others. Yet for every smiling face that would benefit from such efforts, there were many not receiving help. There are over thirty-six million people living in the United States who suffer from food insecurity, and while good things are happening across the nation, there is much work to be done in order to help our fellow Americans.

Our own holiday season would be one filled with warmth and joy as we gathered with our families to share stories, food, and gifts. However, this season had a different ring to it. Our lives had been changed by the dollar-a-day experiment, and as we indulged in larger than necessary holiday portions, we could not forget the extreme hunger we had experienced, nor could we forget those who would be leaning on the community for help.

After celebrating the solstice with my family, for Christmas we drove to Kerri's parents' modest home in Redding, about three hours north of Sacramento. We passed through California's central valley, taking in the fields of fresh produce that make our state the largest farming state in the nation. This four-hundred-mile stretch of flat land is not what people think of when visiting California. Lacking the glamour of Hollywood, sun-soaked beaches, or sites like Disneyland and the Golden Gate Bridge, this quiet part of the state is able to provide 25 percent of our country's food supply. Watching fields of lettuce and strawberries, citrus orchards, and the seemingly endless California aqueduct pass by, I wondered at the amount of food available, and that so many still had to go without.

The ten-hour drive had all but vanished as we pulled into the cul-de-sac around dinnertime. The hearty welcome from Kerri's family reminded me of the value of traditions and the importance of sharing time with loved ones. Throughout the next couple of days, we spent time sitting in the living room and catching up with one another. Staying in our pajamas and not leaving the house, we talked about our lives, read stories to the kids, and waited anxiously for the holiday meal to be ready. People kept arriving, but within no time, all the guests were there and Christmas dinner was served. There was a prayer for Kerri's grandfather, who had been hospitalized for months. Looking around the room, I could see the toll that his decline in health had taken on the family. Christmas wasn't the same without him seated at the head of the table.

As we sat down to eat, I couldn't believe the amount of food laid out before me. There wasn't more than usual for the holidays, but after scraping by on small portions of beans, rice, and peanut butter, this spread resembled a royal banquet. I was overwhelmed by smells of creamy mashed potatoes and spiced stuffing, the clinking of spoons in serving dishes, and the endless stream of bowls that flowed from person to person. In a daze, I nodded as Kerri asked me if I would like some green beans, some potatoes, some bread, some salad. My mind was in a distant land, as if someone had pressed pause on my consciousness. By the time I glanced down, my plate was overflowing with just a little bit of everything. Kerri stared at me and repeated the question she had been asking for the past minute.

"What do you want to drink?"

I snapped out of my trance.

"Water. Water will be fine."

I picked up my fork. I looked down at the helpings in front of me, barely comprehending how all of this food had ended up on my plate. I dipped my fork into the pile of mashed potatoes and looked around to see everyone smiling and enjoying the meal without reservation. Suddenly my mind took me back to September, when a meal like this would have been little more than fantasy. My stomach churned with hunger pangs just thinking about it. I considered the families that would have far fewer options on their tables today. Tasting the lemon-spritzed green beans, I experienced a surge of emotions. The dollar diet taught me about those stabs of hunger that twist a person's insides, and now I sat in the lap of abundance, stunned by the contrast. I did my best to finish the food served to me, but I could not shake those feelings.

We stopped by the Community Resource Center a week later in order to drop off kitchen tools and extra clothes. When we arrived, we saw a line, predominantly made up of women and children who were looking to receive donated food. These were not "freeloaders" who were "too lazy" to get a job and feed themselves; these were the mothers and the children of our community who had fallen on hard times, and who needed just enough help to make it through. Many of the adults had jobs, but still found it hard to feed their families. As we got in the car to head back to the security of our warm house, we remained silent. We knew that there was much more that could be done, and that the dollar-a-day blog was just the beginning of understanding the scope of food issues and hunger in our country. Although the year was coming to an end, we knew that the challenges of unemployment and low incomes would persist beyond the holidays. As people with stable incomes and food security, we had a responsibility to do more.

PART II

THE THRIFTY FOOD PLAN

The Next Challenge

Kerri

The conclusion of our dollar-diet project left us wondering how to better understand the challenges of living with hunger. We had learned that eating on a dollar a day was not enough to have a balanced diet and maintain physical stamina. It even put a strain on our relationship, as tempers ran high and intimacy declined. As people who have always had the means to run to the store without thinking about the cost anytime we needed food, Christopher and I weren't sure we understood what it really cost to eat a healthful diet. But we did know, even before our project, that trips to the market were becoming more and more expensive. If the high cost of groceries created financial strain on us, two high school teachers with moderate incomes, then we knew that the rising costs had to be hitting those living near the poverty line even harder. We wondered whether food assistance programs provided enough relief to low-income families, and whether that relief was enough to ensure a healthy, varied diet. We wanted to know if it was possible for people like the ones we saw waiting in line for food at the Community Resource Center on that rainy evening when we dropped off the donation to eat a diet with sufficient enough fuel to foster productivity at work and home.

It wasn't until we started this experience that I learned that both of my parents had received food stamps for a short time while they were in college. While my family wasn't wealthy, growing up I never felt the insecurity that comes from wondering if there will be enough food in the house. My mom cooked dinner every night, and we always had plenty to eat. After speaking with my parents, I realized how little I knew about food stamps.

When I was in high school, the topic of food stamps somehow came up with two friends. I had no real experience with them, but, as many seventeen-year-olds do, I thought I knew everything. During the course of the conversation, I commented on my frustration with, and silent judgment of, kids who redeemed food stamp dollars for a candy bar or donut. I felt that if their family needed assistance, they should be using it to purchase healthful foods. My friends, whom I did not realize had grown up using food stamps, added their own experiences. They recounted what a huge treat it was to be allowed to go into the store and pick something out on their own. I recalled going to the store with my dad and being allowed to pick out my own candy bar, or our Sunday morning tradition of donuts at the Donut Corner. These moments were special to me, and I soon realized the faulty assumptions I had made about people who received food stamps. I guess I felt that they should only be allowed to eat healthful foods at all times—a standard that I myself didn't want to be held to. I had no idea that these friends of mine had grown up with food stamps; for them, the color-coded tickets were a fact of life.

Several years later, I was in college and working at a grocery store. It was around ten p.m., and the store was pretty empty. I was the only checker, and one manager was on duty. Most likely I was leaning on the counter reading gossip magazines, counting down the hours until I could go home. A woman came up to the counter to make her purchase. When it came time to pay, she pulled out several loose five-dollar food stamp bills. At this time, the electronic benefit transfer cards (EBT), which function like debit cards, did not exist. The rule was that the five- and ten-dollar bills either had to be attached to the booklet they came from, and the checker or customer had to tear them out at the time of purchase, or the customer had to have the booklet with her, and the serial numbers and the stamps needed to match the booklet. To cut down on fraud, we weren't allowed to give five- and ten-dollar food stamp coupons in change, only one-dollar coupons. I have always been the type of person who is nervous to break any rules (Christopher makes fun of me because I *will* keep off the grass if a sign tells me to). So I let the lady know that I would just need to call the manager over to make sure I could take them. She told me that she had been given this as change, and I assured her that it wasn't a big deal, but I wasn't allowed to take them until the manager okayed it.

As soon as I called the manager over, I realized my mistake and wished that I had just taken the bills. In reality, if I had just taken the loose stamps and put them in the till, no one would have known if they had been ripped out right then or not. I explained the situation, and the manager told the woman that we would not be able to take the bills. The woman insisted. She was just trying to get her groceries so that she could go home. She kept looking at me as if I had let her down. I felt horrible, and I couldn't make eye contact with her. The conversation between the customer and the manager kept getting more heated, and I wanted to crawl under my register. A line started to form behind her. Indignant, the woman stated that she wouldn't leave the store until she was allowed to buy her groceries. The manager's solution was to move the people in the line and me to a different register, leaving the woman standing at the counter alone.

After I had checked out the people in the line, I looked up to see that the woman was still standing there. This was when my manager called the police. The whole time, the woman didn't say a word, but stood there, looking down with her hands folded on the countertop. By this point it was obvious that she was shaken, but she quietly waited, clearly trying to maintain her dignity. When the police arrived, they escorted her outside. As they left the store, I heard her saying, "All I did was try to buy food."

I can't imagine how humiliating it must be to be denied this basic human right by a stickler of a college kid and a stubborn store manager. To make matters worse, a few days later, I saw a different manager take unattached five-dollar food stamps without a comment. My shame was palpable, but it no doubt paled in comparison to the embarrassment and frustration the woman felt that evening.

With these as my only experiences with food stamps, I expected this next project to be compelling. Of course, the Food Stamp Challenge is not new. It started with Greater Philadelphia's Coalition Against Hunger in 2006 as a way to demonstrate the struggles of people living on food stamps. Most recently, the challenge of living on food stamps gained attention in May 2007 when Oregon governor Theodore R. Kulongoski ate on twenty-one dollars for one week, which at the time represented the average allotment given to Oregonians in need. Later that same year, several members of Congress took on the same challenge and blogged about their experiences. Typically the person or family participating in the challenge uses only the average per-person allowance, doing their shopping and eating from that amount for a week. In February 2009, CNN reporter Sean Callebs lived off the average food stamp allotment in his home state of Louisiana for an entire month.

When planning our own challenge, Christopher and I arrived at our per-day budget based on the 2007 national average per-person allowance, which at the time was three dollars a day. However, one of the largest criticisms of the Food Stamp Challenge comes from the fact that the program that provides food stamps is now called Supplemental Nutrition Assistance Program (SNAP). The words "Supplemental Assistance," people argue, indicate that the program is not meant to be the entire budget for food. They will also claim that three dollars is not an accurate daily food budget because SNAP assistance is given on a sliding scale based on need; so some families receive more, some receive less. However, just like our dollar-diet project, it would be impossible to accurately mimic every real-life scenario and individual situation, which is why we used the *average* allotment. Also, while it is true that the SNAP program is meant to be supplemental, the reality is that for many people, what they receive in food stamps is all they can afford to spend on food, even though the state assumes they can contribute to their own food budget. The Economic Research Service, a division of the USDA, says that the Social Security Administration estimate in the 1960s, which is still used today, showed that people contribute approximately 30 percent of their disposable income (income after taxes) to food. That is still the system used for calculating need. However, currently the average U.S. household spends less than 10 percent of their income on food, and housing takes up a larger percentage. That 10 percent for a low-income family is not going to go as far as 10 percent for a middle-income family, and the amount of assistance actually needed may not match what people receive.

Because of the belief that people can contribute, and because at the time we conducted our project the stimulus package had also allowed for a temporary 13 percent increase in SNAP benefits, Christopher and I decided that we would contribute 30 percent of a "low-income budget" to food. According to the USDA's April 2007 issue of *Amber Waves* magazine, the average low-income ($10,000–$29,999 per year) household of four in 2004 spent $462 on food per month. By subtracting the national average food stamp benefit, which was $326 per month, we learned that the average supplemented contribution was $136 per month for four people, or $1.13 per day, per person. This gave us $8.26 total or $4.13 each, per day. The Food Stamp Challenge is typically done for one week, but Christopher and I decided to try our thrifty food project for a month. Unlike the dollar-diet project, we would not be purchasing in bulk and calculating only what we ate from our supplies. Instead, for this project we would calculate everything we purchased, limiting our spending to $247.80 for the thirty days.

Another difference was that we would follow the USDA Thrifty Food Plan as closely as possible. The Thrifty Food Plan is supposed to work as a guideline for low-income households to effectively use the SNAP benefits and get the most nutritional value out of the purchased food. The Thrifty Food Plan has admirable intentions. It attempts to assist recipients with creating balanced meals that follow the food pyramid and that can be purchased with the maximum allotment of the SNAP program. The Thrifty Food Plan is not intended to be a strict menu, but rather to help people learn how to make the most out of their resources. According to the "Recipes and Tips for Healthy, Thrifty Meals" put out by the USDA Center for Nutrition Policy and Promotion, the USDA is "deeply concerned that Americans not only have enough food, but also that the public has enough information to know what food to purchase and how to prepare it."

The Thrifty Food Plan provides two weeks' worth of sample menus, forty recipes, and a shopping list. One of the concerns I had about the plan was that it doesn't necessarily list the ingredients in sizes that can be purchased, but rather in the quantity that is needed to make the recipes. Week One on the Thrifty Food Plan includes two ounces of brown sugar, nine ounces of vegetable oil, four ounces of low-salt crackers, and seven ounces of margarine. Obviously, these products can't typically be purchased in those sizes. It was unclear whether the stated cost for the menu is calculated in the same way we calculated our meals for the dollar-diet project, only including what is consumed, or if it takes into account that if you need two ounces of brown sugar, you will most likely need to purchase a twelve- or sixteen-ounce box, or else run next door to see if your neighbor has some. Spices such as onion powder, garlic powder, and Italian seasonings are included in the recipes, but not on the shopping list. It makes sense in that you don't need to buy spices every month, but their cost must be accounted for at some point. We happened to have the spices we needed at home, but if we hadn't, we would have had to either eat bland food or buy them.

Another odd feature of the Thrifty Food Plan are the opening tips for shopping with cost and health in mind. The food plan seems to disregard its own advice: The tips recommend whole wheat bread, brown rice, and dried beans instead of canned, while the recipes include only white bread, white rice, and canned beans.

Despite the fact that this was unclear, we attempted to follow the plan as much as possible. Before we even started, staying on track would prove a challenge for us. The plan is designed to fit the eating preferences of the average American family of four, with two adults and two children between the ages of six and eleven. This makes practical sense; any type of preplanned diet will need to be general enough to be accessible for the largest number of people. Yet Christopher and I don't eat meat or any other animal products, and this food plan was heavy on meat and dairy. Right away, this meant that we would need to make modifications in the menu. Out of the forty recipes, most of the side dishes or snacks are vegetable-based, but only one of the twenty entrees is vegetarian: a baked potato with cottage cheese. I felt that there should have been more options for vegetarian meals in the menu. While we are vegan by choice, there are many people who have restricted diets for other reasons. Some people eat vegetarian for religious reasons, and for others health is the determining factor in what they eat. I am certain that finicky children play a role in family food choices as well.

Christopher and I don't have any kids, besides the furry ones, but I have seen my sisters try to feed my nieces. The girls won't always eat what they are being served. One of my nieces, Leah, the sassy one, went through a phase where she would only eat if you asked her what she wanted. My sister was pretty smart in offering her two options, so she could chose one. This eliminated a guessing game of "What will Leah eat?" and ensured that at least she wouldn't starve.

When Christopher and I take the dogs to visit, though, it may not matter what's being served. The kids tend to eat less because they think it's funny to throw food from their high chairs and watch the dogs eat it—something we try to put a stop to.

The food plan for a family of four assumes that the children are between six and eleven years old. I imagine it is quite different feeding six-year-olds as compared to teenage boys. My brother-in-law is one of four boys who are close in age, all of whom played football in high school. He claims that he never knew what leftovers were until he married my sister, because in his family, there was no such thing.

Regardless of the challenges, we decided to do our best to adhere as closely as possible to the Thrifty Food Plan. Our first task was to plan our meals and grocery list. Many of the meals revolve around some type of ground meat, and the menu includes a glass of milk daily. Because of the large quantity of meat and dairy, before our first shopping trip, I had to modify the recipes and ingredients so that we could follow the plan as closely as we could, getting comparable nutritional value. Also, the recipes were meant to feed a family of four, so we would be making the recipes as they were written, but eating them for two meals instead of one.

Surprisingly, the most frustrating aspect of preparing the menu wasn't having to figure out how to "veganize" the meals. No, the most frustrating part was Christopher. I asked him to help me create a menu for the week, and he told me he was busy. Granted, he was reading about the food stamp system in our country, but I can't imagine how reading about the history of the food stamp system helps when you're trying to figure out what to eat. While reading up on history and policy would help us understand the issue in broader terms, I needed some more concrete immediate help.

"What do you think if I move the turkey-cabbage casserole to Tuesday?" I asked him.

"I don't know" was his response.

"Okay, well, it seems like an easier recipe. Then I could make the potato soup that same night so it would be ready for lunches, but then I'm not sure when to make the meal that's supposed to be on Thursday. That has us eating pasta for lunch and dinner two days in a row. . . . Can you take a look?" I tried again.

He glanced at my menu and then went back to his book. "I don't know. Whatever you want is fine."

"I could really use your help." This was exasperating; my patience was waning.

"I don't know what to do with it." He shrugged.

"What makes you think *I do*?" I tossed my pile of menu revisions onto my desk. I didn't know how to make this work any more than he did. I needed feedback, not a mumbled "Whatever you think." When we did our original project, one reason for my hesitation was that I knew I'd be doing most of the time-consuming cooking. As it is, in general I do most of the meal planning and dinners. Christopher does school lunches and breakfasts, but those tend to be quick. We almost always do our weekly grocery shopping together, but if we need to run back for an item or two during the week, I'm usually the one to go. I don't know why it works out this way, but it just does.

I'm not sure at what point we fell into these conventional gender roles. When we first met, Christopher used to cook for me, and when we moved in together, we took turns, but over the years, I had taken on more of the responsibilities of cooking. In my family, my mom did most of the cooking and on the rare occasions when we ate fast food, it was often when it was my dad's turn to cook. When we get home from work, I'm just as tired as Christopher is, but the first thing he does is read the newspaper, and the first thing I do is start on dinner. Sometimes I enjoy the setup. Christopher will sit at the island in the kitchen and read articles to me while I cook. Some days, though, *I* want to be the one who gets to come home and sit down. I'd like Christopher to be the one planning meals once in a while.

In that moment while I was trying to create the menu, I wanted to cry out in frustration. While Christopher's perception was that he *was* helping by doing research, I felt as if I was doing all the preparation, while he was just reading. He didn't seem to get why I was upset.

There was more to consider than just substituting vegetarian items for nonvegetarian items; I also had to figure out how to manage the prep time. The end of the school year was fast approaching; the entire time I worked on the menu, the stack of my students' essays on the counter haunted me. They had been written over a week earlier, and I had only graded two out of almost eighty.

According to the Thrifty Food Plan, the meals are supposed to be "quick, easy, tasty, and economical," and I hoped they lived up to this expectation. I felt pressed for time as it was, but I wasn't encouraged as I looked over the meals, which conveniently come with estimated preparation and cooking times. Some of the meals that were planned for lunches seemed challenging for people who worked. For example, Friday's lunch is potato soup, which appears nowhere else in the week's menu. It isn't a leftover from another meal, so it needs to be made the day before. When I created our version of the menu, I made a note when we needed to prepare food for the next day. For example, after dinner, or while making dinner on Tuesday, I would need to start cooking baked potatoes to go with lunch on Wednesday. On top of that, because the meal plan is created for a family of four, our daily nutritional values would still be off because we'd be eating quite a few more leftovers than the two-week plan included.

Because we were substituting products, the nutritional value would be different, but we stuck to replacing milk with soymilk and meats with soy and wheat-based alternatives or other proteins such as legumes. Furthermore, we also had to consider the cost. We weren't sure how our milk and meat alternatives would compare to the real thing. We would make it a point during our shopping trip to price-check the products that we didn't purchase (e.g., milk) and compare the prices with products we did purchase (e.g., soymilk), to see how much of a difference it made in our totals. We found that while some of our items were a little more expensive, it wouldn't completely throw off our project. The meat alternatives, such as mock ground turkey and seitan, were comparable in price to the cost of the actual meat, although, on our first shopping trip, we did find soymilk to be more expensive by about a dollar a gallon. We probably could have shopped around to find better prices, but as much as possible we were attempting to go to as few stores as we could. Often people don't have the luxury of being able to spend an afternoon looking for the best price. Then there's the trade-off of running around looking for a bargain, and the cost of gas or bus fare it takes to do so.

Again, we can't pretend that a monthlong experiment is an accurate portrayal of people's experiences. There are many differences between what we were setting out to do and the everyday realities of people living at poverty level. Realistically, Christopher and I could quit anytime, but we also were only experimenting with food. During this month, we wouldn't have to make a decision between eating and paying a bill, a trip to the doctor, or child care. Another big difference between our experience and that of those who actually receive food assistance is that Christopher and I could go through a grocery line without the stigma attached to paying with food stamps or an EBT card. We didn't have to fear that people were looking at how we were paying and then scrutinizing our choices. One of the friends who grew up with food stamps told me that she used to hide at the magazine rack and pretend to read while her mom paid because she was so embarrassed.

It was early evening by the time I conquered the menu. We gathered our shopping bags and headed for the car. I double-checked to make sure my precious list was tucked into my purse. When we started the dollar-diet project, I was full of anticipation. This time I was confident that we would make it through, but I felt anxious about what was in store. "You ready?" Christopher asked as I clicked my seat belt into place. I nodded. He started the car and we headed off.

Strange Combinations

Christopher

Striding through the automatic doors at one of the conventional chain groceries in town, we grabbed a cart and pushed through the immaculate entrance. Having spent a month eating on a dollar a day, we felt confident that with our purchasing power more than quadrupled, we would now be able to live the good life on just over four dollars per day. If we could survive for an entire month on small servings of beans and rice, homemade soups, and tablespoons of peanut butter, this new challenge would be easy. No more itsy-bitsy portions, no more nutritional deprivation, no more monotonous meals. Liberation had arrived. We were looking not just to survive, but to thrive.

As we scanned our USDA-approved shopping list, which seemed longer than any list we had ever made, we rolled the cart over to the produce section. Kerri whipped out her phone calculator: It was time to get down to business. Working out the best deals on cabbage, carrots, potatoes, apples, bananas, oranges, and cantaloupe, we paused to savor the bounty of fresh fruits and vegetables in our cart. I glanced at Kerri and smiled; this meal plan was going to be delicious. I envisioned packing melon slices into Kerri's lunch in the morning and putting some into my own lunch bag as well. However, once we turned down the next aisle, things became more complicated. Staring down the seemingly endless row of boxes and cans while Kerri surveyed the cost per ounce of vegetable oil, my initial eagerness started to fade.

"This bottle is cheaper, but it's way smaller. It doesn't make sense to buy this size, but that's what we can afford on this budget," Kerri complained.

She was right. It made little sense for us to buy things in such small quantities if the next size up offered more value per ounce, but we had no choice. Buying in bulk wasn't an option. It was clear that this project would offer some challenges we hadn't anticipated. While I was excited to push our meal planning to the next level, I started to feel frustrated. Laboring over the cost differences between brands and sizes wasn't something I had been looking forward to, and yet here we were again discussing exactly that. Such conversations were novel during the dollar experiment, but by this point, the mystique had vanished. I just wanted to shop and eat.

Never again would I spend carelessly on food (the dollar-diet project killed that habit), but at this moment, my mind began to fog as the arduous task of counting pennies unfolded before us once again. I could have been doing a ton of other things at this moment that would have been far more productive, and thinking about them only increased my frustration. I could be planning new courses of study for my students. I could be exercising. I could be reading or making lesson plans. Anything would be better than pushing this metal cage on wheels while punching numbers into a calculator for every item on our list. Grocery shopping is not an electrifying experience as is, but having to do it with tough economic restraints made it downright painful. The shopping routines we developed during the first project definitely made things easier, but it did not make things pleasurable.

As we neared the end of the second aisle, more processed items found their way into our cart. Kerri sensed my shopper's fatigue and did her best to remain cheerful, but by the time we hit the cereal aisle, about halfway through the store, an hour had passed. I grabbed a large box of store-brand cornflakes with mild enthusiasm; at least breakfast would be better than before. We still hadn't touched our leftover stash of oatmeal in the cupboard since we ended the previous project.

It was clear, despite our reservations, that this diet would be somewhat more varied. However, in addition to sacrificing bulk values because of our food stamp budget restraints, this plan was already showing another sign of inadequacy. It was difficult to shop for just the two of us on a program constructed for a family of four. Things like the box of cereal in our cart were only available in one size, and no other manufacturer sold a smaller box of cornflakes. We did our best to adjust as we went along, but once we hit the bread section, it was obvious that in some cases, we were better off shopping "off the list" and at our natural foods store instead. After searching for about ten minutes, we found a couple of different loaves we could buy, but both were far too expensive. If I'm going to pay three dollars for a loaf of bread, it might as well be organic and made from whole grains with fewer processed ingredients. The options in front of us were neither healthy nor worth the cost. Luckily for us, we live in an area that boasts several different places to shop; we had options, unlike many in redlined urban areas.

When we reached the checkout, our cart was full of food, and we prepared to spend a large portion of our month's food stamp budget. Since the meal plan and the list were designed for four, this food would have to last at least two weeks, hopefully longer. It dawned on me that this process is what low-income families must do if they are going to effectively feed their families for the month with help from the Supplemental Nutrition Assistance Program. I had read that families who receive this assistance often struggle to make the food last for the entire month, and now I could see why. While there are other government food programs to help our citizens—such as the Women, Infant, and Children (WIC) program, which provides vouchers for particular products, such as frozen orange juice, and the school lunch program—most people in need of assistance from the government do access SNAP.

The food stamp program got its start in 1939 due to a push from industry to help sell particular surplus foods by giving people orange and blue stamps each week. The orange stamps could be used on any food item; for every dollar's worth spent using orange stamps, participants would get back fifty cents' worth of blue stamps, which could only be used on those targeted surplus items. In just a few years, four million people were participating in the program, but as surpluses diminished, so did the support for the program. Farmers alleged that the program was being abused by recipients, and by grocers who would accept the stamps for nonsurplus foods or cash. By 1943, the program was eliminated.

Twenty years later, President Lyndon Johnson launched his war on poverty, and in 1964, after a three-year pilot program in West Virginia, the Food Stamp Act became law and was expanded to many other areas in the Midwest. After a steady number of reports emerged about the hardships of Americans living in economic distress, a CBS television documentary entitled *Hunger in America* highlighted poverty as a national issue. Robert Kennedy toured the South, as did other members of Congress, to see the plight of America's malnourished firsthand. What they saw greatly startled them and moved them to action on the issue. Republican senator Bob Dole and Democrat George McGovern crossed party lines to work together on finding solutions to the nation's poverty epidemic. Throughout the late 1960s and early 1970s, several groups conducted surveys assessing the health of people living in poverty.

Although the validity of some studies was questionable, and the results highly varied based on a number of different factors, one thing was clear: Hunger was indeed a major problem. Children suffered stunted growth and brain damage as a result of malnourishment, and adults became so nutritionally impaired that they could not work. Several nongovernmental hunger organizations sprouted up, and President Richard Nixon held the first and only White House Conference on Food, Nutrition, and Health to address the issue of hunger in America. In 1974 the program went nationwide, and three years later, under President Jimmy Carter, several changes were made, including raising the general resource limit, penalizing heads of households who voluntarily quit their jobs, restricting eligibility for students and nonresidents, eliminating the requirement that households receiving assistance must have cooking facilities, and requiring states to develop disaster plans. The reforms in 1977 ultimately made the program far more accessible and far more efficient.

When these and other changes went into effect in 1979, participation increased by 1.5 million people in the first month alone. Through these efforts, our country helped put an end to the worst cases of hunger in the United States. However, during the era of President Ronald Reagan, the number of Americans facing food insecurity rose significantly. Reaganomics failed to bring wealth to anyone except the already wealthy, and sharp cuts to a slew of social services, including WIC and food stamps, which even included keeping the food stamp program from doing outreach, gave rise to thousands of food pantries and other nonprofit feeding groups nationwide. President Reagan's cuts to social programs, which the Congressional Budget Office estimates at $110 billion from 1982 to 1986, were arguably not the most memorable part of his domestic policy. When his administration tried to cut funding for school lunches by attempting to categorize ketchup as a vegetable, it was so ridiculous that commentators and editorial cartoonists couldn't help mocking the idea.

More changes to the food stamp program were made under President Bill Clinton, and by 1995, the participation rate was at a historic high. In addition, the growing economy allowed many people to walk away from the program altogether. Throughout the Reagan and Clinton administrations, program growth slowed, but in the years that followed, most of President George W. Bush's attempts to cut food stamps failed, and by 2006, participation levels were back up to what they were in the mid-1990s.

Today, SNAP helps bring food to over twenty-nine million people in the United States, and while many people like to think of the average food stamp recipient as a loafer living off the public dole, this stereotype has little evidence to support it. According to the USDA, about half of the participants are children, 76 percent of benefits go to households with children (the majority of which are led by single mothers), 16 percent go to people with disabilities, 9 percent go to elderly persons, and 29 percent earn income through work. And of those who receive benefits, half leave the program in nine months or less; the average recipient participates for less than two years. Additionally, eligibility requirements for SNAP make sure that participation is limited to those who have less than $2,000 in "countable resources," which includes all possible bank accounts, and even something like a car. If your car is worth more than $4,650 in market value, it is part of your countable resources and limits you from receiving aid. If you are an able-bodied person between the ages of eighteen and fifty-five, with no children, you can only receive benefits for ninety days total over a three-year period. The amount of these benefits fluctuates based on a few different factors.

Efforts such as SNAP, WIC, the school lunch program, and other initiatives have moved our nation's impoverished from a state of perpetual hunger to one of food insecurity, which is progress. Before starting this project, I, too, was unsure of just how the food stamp program worked and could do nothing but sit silently as people I knew talked about "those people living off our hard-earned tax dollars." As Kerri and I now waited to be rung up, I wondered how many people had come through this line today ready to use their EBT cards to buy groceries. Once the clerk scanned all of our items, the total came to just over $117, a little less than half of our monthly budget. On the way home from the store that evening, it was clear that this was not going to be as easy as we had thought.

The next morning was our first breakfast on the Thrifty Food Plan experiment, and we were pleasantly surprised by the change from the dollar diet. I opened the cornflakes and scooped three-quarters of a cup into my little white bowl, dropped the English muffins into the toaster, and opened the door of the fridge to pull out the orange juice. Even though we still had to measure our portions, the fact that they were far larger and more palatable made it less of a bother than before. When Kerri emerged from the bathroom, I measured out the soymilk and dumped it into her bowl. Crunching through cornflakes felt great. There is nothing like relishing the flavor of this sweet American ritual, especially if you haven't had them in years. The English muffin sat waiting for me to chew through its toasted goodness, and the orange juice made for a smooth chaser.

I took a look at the menu to start preparing lunch: turkey burgers, coleslaw, and more orange juice. I wasn't sure how to approach this new change in packing lunches; it took much longer than I had time for. Surely they didn't expect working people to have the time on their lunch breaks to stop and cook up a burger or chop cabbage for slaw. Kerri finished her breakfast a few minutes later and started to work on making the coleslaw as I pulled the vegan chicken patties, our substitute, from the freezer.

Kerri very rarely had to help me make lunches on normal mornings, but there was a time or two when the alarm failed to go off and Kerri pinch-hit for me. Today the clock was ticking. I grabbed a couple of hamburger buns and dug around in the top shelf of the refrigerator door to find some leftover ketchup packets from a previous visit to Rico's. I threw the burgers in the Foreman grill and shortly afterward put them in the buns and sealed our lunches in small containers.

Kerri had finished making the coleslaw and was measuring out our servings and packing them up. I had never liked coleslaw and wasn't sure if her efforts would be worth the trouble if I couldn't bring myself to eat the stuff. This extra time spent preparing lunch had already put me fifteen minutes behind for work. I couldn't be bothered to figure out how to transport three-quarters of a cup of orange juice with me to school as the meal plan stated, so I drew an arrow from the orange juice down to the "Snack" section. We could drink it after work. Besides, we had used our only pitcher to make the orange juice, so the proposed lemonade in the plan wouldn't be happening just yet. Behind schedule and ready to leave, I made a mental note to make sure that this wouldn't happen again tomorrow. I had appointments with students every ten minutes starting at seven a.m., and being even a minute late would push everyone back and make the start of my first class even more stressful.

At lunchtime I gave my burger a quick zap in the microwave and, after dutifully enjoying every moment of it, I opened up the coleslaw and dared to take a bite. I lifted the shredded cabbage and carrot mixture to my lips, my nose crinkling as the vinegar dressing coated my tongue. Actually, it wasn't terrible. The half-cup serving was gone in no time, and I found myself licking the dressing from the sides of the plastic container. Was I really doing this? I'd spent my whole life avoiding the dish at family get-togethers, and during my previous fast-food life, it was the only container still full at the end of one of the KFC meals that other people's parents picked up for dinner. Lunch left me feeling satisfied, but I wondered for how long. Usually when I get home from work, I need an after-school snack—a habit that still lingers from my elementary school days.

By the time I got home, I was surprised to see Kerri there; usually I arrived before her. Walking into the kitchen, I saw that she had already prepared the prescribed snack option from the plan for that day: chickpea dip. Despite the fact that she had followed the recipe provided by the Thrifty Food Plan, the dip wasn't what I expected. When I see things like "chickpea dip," the foodie in me thinks: hummus. This was not the case. The gritty consistency was a far cry from the smooth lather that I had become accustomed to in Middle Eastern restaurants and store-bought brands. I spread the concoction over a slice of bread and took a bite; not bad. I poured myself the ration of juice that had been meant for lunchtime, and asked Kerri, "So what's for dinner?"

She inspected the meal plan and raised her eyebrows.

"Beef noodle casserole, lima beans, banana and orange salad, and half a cup of milk."

"That's a strange combination," I commented.

Before dinner we went over the Thrifty Food Plan menu, and I saw how Kerri had decided to mix up some of the offerings, as we would end up having enough leftover casserole that evening for lunch the following day. Moreover, there was no way I would have been able to prepare the crispy chicken for lunch. The recipe was far too complex for the amount of time I had in the morning. In order to make it before work, I would have had to get up at four thirty a.m., an hour earlier than usual. I could have prepared the vegan equivalent that night, but Kerri would be busy making dinner, and our kitchen isn't built with lots of counter space, nor do we have enough dishes for two people to develop large meals simultaneously.

The reorganizing of the meal options was an absolute necessity because otherwise our fridge would be bursting with leftovers, and because the time allotted for preparing lunches is totally unrealistic for working people. We wondered if this plan was developed for the stay-at-home parent, or if the USDA was encouraging working less so you could stay home and play domestic engineer. Adjusting the menu made it difficult to guarantee that we were still eating in line with the food pyramid. We did our best to modify things in order to ensure that we were getting the prescribed amount of protein, calcium, whole grains, fruits, and vegetables each day.

However, as the week wore on, we noticed that many of the meals started to taste the same. Lots of casseroles, lots of pasta, lots of meat and dairy, and of course the daily regimen of orange juice. Snacks like biscuits, dips, and pasta salads were peppered throughout the week, but Kerri was already beginning to grow weary of the plan.

For me, things were great. I loved the saucy beef pasta and the turkey cabbage casserole. I rejoiced over my morning juice and nightly half-cup of soymilk with dinner; it reminded me of my childhood, when milk with dinner was mandatory. The meals were a strange journey into my earlier eating life, and much like visiting an old familiar place, I felt a welcome note in every bite. The only mildly challenging experience for me was the cooked rice cereal. Traditionally, rice is something you eat as a side dish with dinner, and maybe sometimes in pudding. Even that was rare, considering I've only had rice pudding three times in my entire life. I couldn't see rice as a breakfast food unless it came with three little elves named Snap, Crackle, and Pop. After a gloopy month of oatmeal, the prospect of another mushy breakfast was not appealing. Cooked with milk and flavored with sugar and cinnamon, this hot porridge was edible, but thankfully it appeared in the plan only once that week. We could cope.

9

Confessions

....

Kerri

When I worked at a grocery store—where I made over minimum wage, got two weeks of paid vacation, sick leave, and medical, dental, and vision insurance—I often worked until ten or eleven p.m., but my schedule changed every week. This would leave me little time to plan or prepare meals. On evenings when I ended work late, I would grab fast food from a nearby restaurant on the way home. Exhausted, having been on my feet most of the day, the last thing I wanted to do was make dinner. In my job now, although I'm also on my feet for hours, I'm not pushing carts or doing any heaving lifting. Still, I'm tired when I get home and have to muster the energy to make dinner.

Christopher and I enjoyed our free time on Sunday. In fact, at six p.m., I awoke from a forty-five-minute nap on the "magic couch," so named because it is impossible to read on it without falling asleep. I rolled off the couch and wandered into the kitchen to prepare dinner. I reached for the box of bowtie pasta stored in the cupboard and discovered that we had only about one cup of pasta left, while the meal I had planned to make called for 6 3/4 cups. We had eaten a late breakfast and skipped lunch, as we tend to do on the weekends, so when dinnertime rolled around, we were ready to eat.

"Guess what?" I groaned to Christopher. "We need to go to the store."

"Really?" he asked. "Is there anything we can make instead?"

"I'll look," I said, "but I doubt it."

The problem was that we couldn't just run out for pasta. We also needed to consider what else we required for the week so (in theory) we would not have to go again. After almost forty-five minutes of digging through the pantry to see if we could substitute ingredients, poring over the Thrifty Food Plan, and exchanging a few tense words about whether or not we were meeting the nutritional guidelines for a balanced diet every day (we were not), we set out for the store.

On a tip from a friend, we went to a different store than we had on our first shopping trip. Upon hearing where we went the first time, Spencer claimed that another store, which thankfully happened to be closer to our house, would have cheaper prices. He was right: We could have saved a few dollars if we had shopped there in the first place. I was surprised by the deals in the pasta aisle. I could buy ten bags of pasta for ten dollars. I was equally in awe of how inexpensive junk food was. A large end-cap display held two-liter soda bottles, also ten for ten dollars. As we walked by, several people were taking advantage of this sale.

We made our way through the store as quickly as possible with our rumbly tummies guiding the way, but this "quick" shopping trip dragged on longer than our patience could handle. We needed to run to another store for a few items that we couldn't get at the first one. On the way home, we stopped at a third store so I could run in and get a cheap pitcher, since we needed another one for the plan. By the time we got home and made dinner, we had spent another $43.79, and it was nine p.m. before we finally sat down to eat. The most frustrating part about this experience was the fact that there was no one to blame but ourselves. We had planned poorly.

During the dollar-diet project, one phenomenon that surprised me was that our refrigerator always seemed full of food, but we were eating so little. Of course that food lasted us for several meals, and we did much of our preparation for the week during the weekend. Likewise, in the second week of this phase, I had noticed that we again had a full fridge. Because of our small portions, plenty of leftovers remained. There was a container holding the remains of a can of peaches, leftover casserole from Sunday, a partial container of orange juice, a carton of soymilk, a head of cabbage (neither of us liked cabbage, but as it was an ingredient in a couple of recipes, we agreed to give it a shot).

On our shopping trip that evening, we purchased some of the ingredients for the menu for the second week on the Thrifty Food Plan, but not all of them. Again, due to the fact that there were two of us—not four—we needed to make our food last longer. For now it seemed as if there was an abundance of food in our fridge, but we realized that we needed to make it last. Because we were supplementing the SNAP average ($3 per person each day) with our own funds ($1.13 per person each day), we still had $90.41 remaining in our food budget for the month, in addition to the food in our cupboards to get us through the next couple of weeks. However, had we not been able to supplement, and had to spend only $180 for the month (an average allotment for two people), we would have had only $20.90 remaining.

The meals recommended by the plan aren't bad. Again, I longed for a little more variety than Christopher did, but we both warmed to the menus. The initial three recipes I made had the same first two steps: Chop onions, then sauté with either ground turkey or ground beef. One recipe required tomato sauce, another required a can of tomato soup poured over it, and they all used either pasta or rice. The recipes lived up to the promise of being easy to make, but they weren't always fast, and I wondered about how healthy they were. Most of the ingredients were inexpensive, and it made sense to simplify shopping by incorporating similar ingredients into several different recipes to minimize waste. I was happy with the inclusion of produce, but we were eating far more in the way of pasta and meat substitutes than we typically do. Our main fruits and vegetables included oranges, orange juice, canned pears or peaches, and green beans. It was better than not having fruits and veggies at all, and despite the lack of variety, we were much more satisfied after eating these meals than on our dollar budget.

Because our new budget was over four times more than that of our dollar diet, and given the fact that we weren't focusing on our daily totals as much as our total cost, Christopher and I both felt like we could "get away" with more. Early in our second week, I left my water bottle at home. Around the end of second period, my work period, I was snacking on my lunch and needed something to wash it down. The nearest water source to my classroom is a bathroom; I had no intention of getting water from there. I have a little change container in my top desk drawer, so I counted out its contents to see if I had enough for a soda from the teachers' room. I had forty-five cents. That wouldn't get me very far. I dug out my wallet and shook out the change. It rained nickels and dimes. As I counted it into my hand, I debated whether or not I should actually use it. After all, we were supplementing with $1.13 per day, but I wasn't sure if I wanted to spend half of that on a soda. Not to mention the fact that there is too much sugar and no nutritional value in soft drinks, and I typically prefer my caffeine in the form of coffee. Of course, I rationalized this by comparing it to the $1.25 it would have cost to get a bottle of water from a different vending machine. The cheaper option didn't seem like the best choice, but I decided that one soda wouldn't blow the whole experience.

One thing I did worry about was what I would say to Christopher. I would need to tell him something to explain why seventy-five cents had been added on from nowhere. I started having flashbacks to the cookie argument during September that could have ended our relationship (or just left us pissed off for the day). I worried, too, about opening the floodgates: If I have a soda today, will I want one tomorrow? Twice I thought about turning back, but I made excuses. I had to go down to the copy machine anyway—the teachers' room is on the way; not only would it cost $1.25 for a bottle of water, but that machine might eat my money (which it is known to do), and that would leave me still thirsty and $1.25 poorer. Then I went for it.

As soon as the ice-cold can dropped into the tray, I felt guilty—it was as if I was stealing food from Christopher. But as I cracked open the can, tipped it back, and felt the cool bubbling sensation on my tongue, there was no more guilt. I swallowed the first gulp and enjoyed every drop.

Several times during the afternoon, I thought about how I would break it to Christopher. I decided to play up the fact that I was thirsty and in need of a drink, while playing down the fact that I made a poor nutrition choice. When I got home, Christopher was on his computer. We chitchatted for about twenty minutes before he decided to get dinner started (i.e., reheating what I had made the night before), and I finally confessed my transgression. I was relieved when he said that it was no big deal. I felt I was off the hook. Seconds later, he confessed that he had been snacking all week on the oatmeal cookies that he had made for one of our meals, and now there were none left for our lunches. While his cookies had to be made as part of the Thrifty Food Plan, they wouldn't cost us more, but the mutual admission of sneaking food was enough to keep both of us watching each other from then on.

When I reminded Christopher that I would be going to my school's play on Thursday night, his first response was, "What will we have for dinner?" I told him that he'd have to be responsible for cooking, which was translated into him heating up leftovers, as it often does on nights when Christopher cooks. The problem became that the leftovers were supposed to be lunch on Friday, and without a new meal prepared, we were left with pathetic lunches. Friday morning turned into a scramble to figure out what to eat. In the end, I sliced up some cabbage for coleslaw, and Christopher packed up grapes and tossed an apple into each of our lunch bags. That day I couldn't complain about not having fruits and veggies in our diet, but it did leave me less than full. I was frustrated by the lack of forethought we had put into planning our meal the night before, and I was annoyed that if I wasn't the one to cook, then little cooking would take place.

When I got home on Friday, I was tired and hungry. I walked into the house to find Christopher snacking on a bag of barbecue-flavored sunflower seeds. We had purchased these prior to starting the Thrifty Food Plan, but, since they weren't given to us, we had to calculate them into our total as well. That was another ninety-nine cents poorly spent. While I was disappointed at the use of our money, I wasn't shy in partaking of the treat. If we both had to pay for it, I might as well enjoy it, too.

That wasn't all I had to look forward to that evening. I was hungry, but excited that I didn't need to cook that night. For this project, we decided that we would take free food whenever it was available, and that night we were going to get a full meal. We were headed to a free weekend conference called "Cultivating Food Justice." As it tied in so nicely with what we were trying to learn about, we were eager to attend. The conference was organized entirely by volunteers in the San Diego area, including San Diego Food Not Lawns, Seeds at City, the California Food and Justice Coalition, San Diego Sustainable Roots, and the International Rescue Committee. The conference would have guest speakers and sessions devoted to food justice issues facing Californians and those in the rest of the United States. Included with the conference was free dinner on Friday night, provided by eleventh and twelfth graders in a culinary arts program at a local high school, and free breakfast and lunch on Saturday, provided by a San Diego chapter of Food Not Bombs.

Despite the fact that we had been talking about issues related to food for months, I wasn't entirely familiar with the phrase "food justice," and I wasn't sure what this conference would be like. When Christopher and I arrived at City College in San Diego, we followed the hand-painted signs and arrows that pointed us to the cafeteria-style room where the keynote speakers would be. We registered and took the bowls and silverware that we brought from home and got in line. Dinner included vegetarian chili, bread, and a garden salad. After having had such a small lunch earlier in the day, I couldn't wait to dig in. We loaded up our bowls and took seats near the front of the room. I greedily ate my chili, but not wanting to take advantage of the hospitality of the organizers, I didn't have a second bowl. I did, however, let Christopher go back and get a second slice of bread for me.

According to the program, "Food justice means that everyone must have access to safe, nutritious, and culturally appropriate food in sufficient quantity and quality to sustain a healthy life with full human dignity." While we ate, I looked around the room, curious about what type of people would attend such a conference. I wanted to see who the people were who believed in this issue. There were several college-aged kids helping to serve the meal and a few more scattered throughout the audience, but there didn't seem to be more of any particular age group than another. There were people who appeared to be my parents' and grandparents' ages, along with the high school students who stayed after the meal to hear the speakers.

Due to Los Angeles traffic, the first speaker arrived a few minutes late. While we waited, one of the organizers put in a documentary called *The Garden* about the fight for the community farm in South Central L.A. When our speaker Rufina Juarez arrived, we learned that she had been instrumental in creating the community farm documented in the film, and eventually the farm that replaced it. She spoke passionately about the needs of her community. Many of the issues were ones that seemed to be themes for the weekend. There is a belief that people in poverty need food, but that quality food is only for people who can afford it. She spoke of the illusion of choice when we go to the grocery store. While we believe we are making decisions about what to put in our baskets, Juarez argued, we don't have control over what is available to us. "Somebody else is making that choice for you," she asserted, referring to the food industry. The community farm she helped to start was eventually evicted from their location in South Central and they relocated to Bakersfield. The farm's eighty acres have up to three thousand visitors on Saturdays, and provide approximately thirty tons of food a year. That food is taken to the South Central Farmers Market, which is one of the only sources of fresh quality food in the area.

The next speaker, LaDonna Redmond, is a community activist from Chicago who got involved in food issues when her child was diagnosed with severe food allergies. Redmond has been instrumental in working to get junk food out of schools in her area and developing urban agriculture. She echoed Juarez's commentary on the lack of choice in our food system, and went a step further to attack the myth that people won't choose to buy fresh food if it is available and affordable. Christopher and I had learned before about "food deserts," areas where there are no grocery stores with healthy food available. These tend to be areas with several liquor stores or small corner markets that may have a few groceries, but at a higher price than a supermarket charges. Redmond looked at these areas differently. She preferred the term "food apartheid" because it better described the system. We left that evening with quite a bit to think about, and five zucchini from a box marked "free."

The following morning, as we ate our provided toast and jam, we listened to that morning's speaker, Malaki Obado Ogendi, discuss traditional agriculture in his home country of Kenya. He ended by giving us tips for working communally: start at home, involve the young, make it social and fun, share knowledge and produce, and make informed choices.

After the speakers, the attendees broke up to attend small group sessions. Christopher and I went to a session called Nutritional Racism. I was surprised to learn that one of the factors used for predicting overall health is the zip code of a person's residency. Poor communities tend to be located near freeways, factories, and waste. It is more likely that the sidewalks and parks are not kept up, and food apartheid is most prevalent in poor communities. In our neighborhood, we have four health food stores within a few miles of one another. Aside from those, there are several major chain grocery stores throughout our town. Our city also has many parks for people and dogs. Conversely, poor communities may not have parks or walking trails for people to get exercise, let alone the money for gym memberships. If there are trails in the neighborhood, it may not be safe to walk for exercise. Christopher and I belong to a gym that I often say we "donate" our money to. Like many people, we will get motivated and go several times a week for a month or so, and then as soon as we get busy or distracted, exercise is one of the first things to go.

When we were in the session, we were asked what we thought were indicators of ill health. I had no idea, and Christopher had guessed stress. This was high in the factors that we discussed in our session. While everyone experiences stress in their lives, people living near the poverty level may have a higher level of stress. On top of the typical stressors of work and family, there may be the added stress of whether or not a bill can be paid. There is also food insecurity: The concern about where the next meal is coming from, or if there will be a next meal, can definitely heighten anxiety. During the dollar project and the thrifty food project, despite the fact that we might not have been eating enough, or *what* we wanted to eat, we still knew that at least we would be eating something. Even so, we were far more stressed than we were when we weren't limiting our food budget. We walked out of that session discussing the privileges that we have.

As we waited in line for our Food Not Bombs lunch, we relished the near-festival atmosphere of the conference. Under the shade of a tree was a woman teaching people how to make canned jams and jellies. Two kids wrestled with their dad, climbing on him like a jungle gym. Another area was covered in cardboard boxes and foil, where people learned how to make their own solar cookers. But the main event happened right in front of us. Out of nowhere, a troop of people dressed as produce pranced out to a central area and began to sing and dance. They sang about the importance of eating fruits and vegetables, but I think my favorite song was about produce having to travel great distances to arrive on your plate, illustrated by a carrot wearing a beret. We got our vegetable and barley soup and a couple slices of bread, and sat under a tree to watch the end of the singing vegetable show.

We only had time for one more session that day, and it was the one that was most helpful for our understanding of our project. It was titled "Bottom of the Barrel: Why does San Diego have the worst food stamp participation in the entire country, and what can we do to change it?"

I knew that California had the lowest food stamp participation in the country, but I didn't know that San Diego had the worst participation in California. According to the workshop, the state's participation rate is 50 percent. This means that of all the people in California who would qualify for food stamps, 50 percent do not apply for or receive them, for whatever reason. In San Diego, at the time of the conference, the participation rate was 30 percent.

While there are numerous reasons why so few eligible people receive benefits, one issue that was discussed was the fact that in order to receive benefits, it isn't uncommon for people to have to visit the office an average of five times, with each visit averaging one hour, in order to get signed up and approved. These visits often mean time off from work, sometimes without pay. The appointments are scheduled at the convenience of the office, not the recipient, and the recipient can only meet with his or her own caseworker. If the caseworker is sick or out of work for any reason, the recipient has to wait for him or her to return before any issues can be addressed. This may cause a delay in receiving or continuing benefits. Another deterrent is the fact that California is one of only a few states that also require fingerprinting before benefits are granted. The reason behind this is to prevent fraud, but it is costly and has done little to make a difference.

Maybe I have seen too many courtroom dramas, but I tend to associate fingerprinting with criminal activity. And while I understand wanting to prevent fraud, the cost of running the fingerprinting program is more than what is saved by preventing fraud. The program requires that everyone over eighteen in a household receiving SNAP benefits must be fingerprinted. The rate of fraud is estimated to be 2 percent. While doing our project, obviously Christopher and I didn't have to go through the humiliating process of being fingerprinted. Nor did we have to spend hours filling out paperwork or taking time away from our jobs to go to the food stamp office. It seems that there are many obstacles to overcome to get assistance to feed your family.

As I've mentioned before, stigma is attached to food stamps. People make assumptions about why people need them. Often the first assumption is that the people in need are lazy. Just like in every situation in life, there will always be a select few who try to take advantage of the system, but the majority of the people receiving benefits depend on them for survival. The program requires that: "All able-bodied persons (ages 18–49) without dependents must work 20 hours per week (monthly average 80 hours), or participate 20 hours per week in an approved work activity or do workfare, or else get only 3 months of Food Stamps out of a 36-month period."

Furthermore, some assume that people could eat healthfully if they wanted to, or if they were educated about how to eat better. While for some people this may be the case, there are many situations where education doesn't matter if healthy options aren't available or affordable. SPIN, the Supportive Parents Information Network in San Diego, a nonprofit, volunteer-run program that works to help families in need, has conducted studies that show that people tend to eat more healthfully at the start of the month. As the money runs out, the meals become less healthful. Additionally, parents report frequently skipping meals so that their children may eat.

One part of the issue that isn't always considered is how increased participation in the SNAP program can support the community. It is estimated that for every $1 in food stamps spent, at least another $1.73 goes into the economy. If food stamps get people to a store, they are more willing to spend other money there as well. In addition, if they have food stamps, they may not have to make a choice between food and bills or medicine.

On the way to the car after the conference, we left feeling hopeful. Many of those in attendance were dedicated to making fresh, healthy food available to everyone, regardless of their economic situation. It was at the conference that we learned about some of the ways people are involved in making change. Specifically, we became interested in the farmers market and plans for a community farm in City Heights, the area of San Diego most in need of assistance. We were stunned to find out that when it comes to food insecurity and providing people with access to food, San Diego is the worst in the nation.

Christopher and I decided to visit the farmers market in City

Heights, to see the efforts being made there. Through collaboration between the San Diego Chapter of the International Rescue Committee and the San Diego Farm Bureau, every week several local farmers bring their produce to City Heights. Right away, it was apparent that this farmers market differed from the one we are used to visiting. Ours is held at a local elementary school and has a wide variety of vendors and booths. In addition to fresh produce, you can purchase everything from crafts to fresh bread to addictive garlic spread. There is usually someone playing live music to the legions of locavores. The City Heights market has a central location: On one corner is the police station, on another is the community college that offers free adult education classes. The community center and library are across the street, and on the opposite side are two low-income housing buildings and a community garden.

There are significantly fewer vendors, as this market is relatively new, and that day there weren't many customers. However, as we walked past the booths, we saw fresh greens stacked up and boxes of vegetables. One vendor had long, slender, vibrant purple eggplants and dark green zucchinis at least a foot long. What I first thought was a place for bike parking was a group of young punk rock volunteers teaching people how to rebuild and repair bikes. But that wasn't why we went.

A table underneath a white canopy stood at the far end. There was a laptop, a wireless card-swiping machine, a group of volunteers in colorful City Heights farmers market T-shirts, and a sign that said: "Use your EBT card here!!!"

EBT cards (which have replaced the food stamp coupons) are swiped in exchange for tokens that can be used at any time at the farmers market. It is rare even to find a farmers market in a low-income area, let alone one that accepts EBT. In addition to helping people who already receive benefits, the San Diego IRC has volunteers helping to prescreen people to find out if they qualify for the SNAP program and fill out initial paperwork for their application. Their volunteers speak Spanish, Vietnamese, and Somali.

According to Andrea Magee, an employee with the IRC, City

Heights has the lowest participation rate in San Diego. This booth was one of the busiest at the time we arrived. As we waited in line to talk to someone, an older woman came up to find out why there were so many people crowded around, and learned that she might qualify for a one-time senior voucher. Two women, one of whom helped to translate, assisted a Somalian man. No one was turned away as the volunteers explained the processes and helped people with their questions. While we waited, we noticed a survey asking customers how the market's prices compared to those at the grocery store. Most of the feedback indicated that the prices were "similar" or "better." When we spoke with two of the workers, we learned that they do surveys every week to better serve their customers and vendors.

This particular market is able to offer what they call "Fresh Funds." Money is donated to the program and is distributed each week, so that people who spend five dollars at the market get an additional five dollars' worth of tokens to spend there. Incentives like this encourage people to use their money on fresh fruits and vegetables while helping local farmers. While there are other farmers markets that accept EBT, they are the exception. There is still an attitude across income levels that farmers markets are for people with money.

After our experience at City Heights, Christopher and I were ready to make our money go further. We weren't necessarily eating as inexpensively as possible because we were staying close to the Thrifty Food Plan. By the end of the second week, we had spent $198.09 out of our $247.80 budget. We still had plenty of food at home, and $49.51 left to make it the next two weeks. If we had been eating only on the food stamp average, we would have already overspent by $18.09. If we hadn't been trying to follow the plan, we could have found ways to eat less expensive foods, and might have had more money left over.

Food Fight

Christopher

With only six weeks of the school year left, the pressure was on to help students prepare for finals, get the last couple issues of the student newspaper out, and wrap everything else up in time for summer. The end of the school year is both a time of great stress and great relief, as it is challenging to manage the progress of 150 students all heading for the finish line. In addition to advising both the journalism and social justice programs, I could feel summer coming, and as the final days grew closer, the heat in my students grew as well.

By the third week of the experiment, we had pretty much figured out how to work within the USDA's plan, but working with each other proved a little more daunting. Kerri was sprinting to close the school year. While students stress about grades and finishing assignments, we teachers work extra hours to provide support for them, leaving less patience for one another. After being flexible all day for students, problem solving at home—especially for mundane things like cooking and laundry—was nearly impossible. There were times when the added stress elicited rolled eyes and snippy comments in the kitchen as we struggled to follow the Thrifty Food Plan. While our experience at the Food Justice conference was both enlightening and motivational, the reality of working as public school teachers made everything a touch more difficult during the week.

It was only Tuesday, but for both of us, it felt as if we had been working all week; we were exhausted. Kerri looked at the menu: crispy chicken, lima beans, and canned peaches. Having adjusted the menu to allow for leftovers, we turned one of the lunch options into a dinner dish. The only problem was that we were out of seitan, our cheap go-to meat alternative. The recipe instructed that you bread the chicken in a seasoned flour mixture and then roll the pieces in cornflakes before baking and eating with barbecue sauce. I was actually looking forward to the dish, but one thing I never look forward to is running out to the store to pick up ingredients after having been at work all day. We had misjudged part of our shopping and left out this key ingredient.

"Could you go to the store?" Kerri asked.

I continued staring at my book.

"Hello?"

I had no interest in putting my shoes back on and getting in the car to run a grocery errand. For the record, I didn't want Kerri to have to go, either. Kerri was pissed. Even though I knew it wouldn't fly, I tried one of my usual excuses.

"I'm in my underwear."

Kerri stared in utter amazement at the banality of my response.

"Oh, really?" she asked.

"Yeah."

Before I could turn to defend my position, Kerri had kicked off her shoes and was in the process of unbuttoning her work pants.

"You don't have to do that," I offered.

"Apparently I do! Whenever we need something from the store, I'm always the one who has to go and get it!" she said.

In a matter of seconds, she had leveled the playing field by stripping down to her undies. She had made her point, and no overtures to the contrary would save me.

"All right, I'll go," I capitulated.

Her disbelief at my indolence was clear, so I pulled on some jeans and made for the door before things got any worse.

ON MY DRIVE to the store, I thought about how lucky we were to live in an area where we had the option to shop without too much hassle, how we had the luxury to choose which store to shop at, and how we were fortunate enough to have a car. Unlike those living in locations where food apartheid is the reality, we were indeed lucky. I parked in front of Jimbo's, grabbed the shopping bag, and headed inside. I hoped that my making the run would ease the situation back home.

A woman in front of me plopped her infant into a shopping cart, and I paused to give her a moment to get through the entrance. She pushed her baby and cart through the automatic doors, and at that moment I thought of something that I had never fully considered before. Shopping carts, in addition to helping customers collect items, evolved with mothers in mind. What started as a place for food became a place for a baby as well. The original shopping cart was invented by Sylvan Goldman in 1936 and looked more like a folding chair with room for two wire baskets, one above and one below. Women scoffed at the idea initially, as it felt too much like a baby carriage. However, just in time for the baby boomers, the shopping cart evolved.

I watched the woman put her purse in the part of the cart closest to her and continued thinking about the division of labor within the home. When I was a child, my mom did most of the cooking and cleaning, and it seemed like the only time I saw a man putting together a meal was outside, at the grill. The tradition of women working in the kitchen and serving the family is one that has developed and changed over time, but after the contributions made to the war effort during World War II, any post-wartime independence for women was publicly discouraged. Women were reminded that their place to be creative was in the home. In a speech titled "The Women in Your Lives," Marjorie Husted, the creator of Betty Crocker, explained to advertisers that women should feel that "a homemaking heart gives her more appeal than cosmetics, that good things baked in the kitchen will keep romance far longer than bright lipstick." The popular belief was that women should not work outside the home, and that those who didn't "had a more interesting time" than those who did.

As women's roles evolved, with more women working outside the home, the responsibility to cook for the family didn't evolve into a shared responsibility. Women now had to work *and* prepare meals for the family. This crunch for time gave food processors the perfect opportunity to create meals that were prepackaged, canned, and frozen in order to meet the needs of women who worked both inside and outside the home.

I knew of this struggle firsthand. After my parents divorced, my mom still cooked quite a bit, but she also had to work during the day and go to classes at night to finish her degree, which meant that the meals were more often boxed macaroni and cheese and canned soup than the homemade pot pies from before they split. My sister and I spent every other weekend at my father's house, and as stated earlier, we ordered pizza or went to a local restaurant. We didn't complain, as these were the few times we were able to eat out, but the difference between how each of our parents provided for us was quite distinct. I wondered if the woman in front of me was in a similar situation.

As I made my way to the back of the store to pick up the seitan, I couldn't help but notice that most of the shoppers around me were women. The worn-out notion that "a woman's place is in the kitchen" should have come with a complementary addendum like "and the grocery store."

This wasn't the first time I had reflected on the disparities between the sexes. Growing up in the punk scene during high school, my introduction to feminism and questioning gender roles came in the form of groups like Bikini Kill, folk singers like Ani Difranco, and the lyrics of male-fronted bands like Good Riddance and Snapcase, who screamed for the equality of women. The ideas took root quickly, and I have considered myself a feminist ever since.

That week in my social justice class, a group of students were working on a case study exploring the current status of the women's movement. One of the young women in the group had asked, "What types of things do you think we should look into?"

I offered up some of the old standbys that still held some power: a woman's right to choose, equal pay, and sexual discrimination. I even suggested that they take a more global look at these issues and study the gender dynamics in places like Afghanistan and Iran—which I thought would expand their discussion of the issues a little bit. However, while helping them develop their ideas on types of questions to ask during their inquiry, I realized that I had some of my own searching to do. In my past relationships, I tried to keep on equal footing with my partners, especially when we started to slip into more traditional roles.

Yet I was letting Kerri take on the bulk of the work at home. How had we relapsed so easily into this patriarchal tradition? How could I change this? These questions had obvious answers. I just needed to repeat what I did in earlier relationships: to do my share of the work and stay vigilant about not exploiting my partner. This included running to the store to pick up the odd grocery item when needed.

I returned home with the necessary supplies, a renewed sense of responsibility, and a growing concern for those women, many of whom are single parents, who work all day and still need to receive federal assistance to feed themselves and their children. When I set the groceries on the counter, I was pleased to see that Kerri had put on some pajama pants and had a forgiving look in her eyes.

The rest of the week was a blur of casseroles and tomato-based dishes, punctuated by a turkey chili served over macaroni that Kerri actually enjoyed. Luckily I had grabbed enough zucchini at the conference to help us prepare a couple of meals, and one night we fried up the green freebies and enjoyed them with biscuits.

By Saturday, the cupboards were starting to look pretty bare, but we weren't yet at a crisis point. In fact, I felt comfortable enough with our newly developed low-cost eating skills that I pulled a couple of cans from the cupboard to place in a bag to put out by the mailbox for the nationwide "Stamp Out Hunger" day. This annual event, the largest one-day national food drive, is sponsored by the National Association of Letter Carriers, and takes place on the second Saturday in May. Close to ten thousand cities in all fifty states participate, and the food collected is distributed within each respective community. In 2009, while unemployment crept to 9.5 percent, and one in nine Americans received SNAP benefits, a record 73.4 million pounds of food was collected through this event.

As I put the canned mandarin oranges and organic tomato sauce in the bag, I wondered about whether or not efforts like this, while commendable in their own right, were part of a greater policy push to end hunger in the United States, or just another drop in the food basket. We had seen the work done by volunteers and the Community Resource Center firsthand, we had given the $2,300 in donations from our readers to help support their food programs, and it felt good to be part of an effort to help those suffering from food insecurity—but was it actually helping? As I watched for the mail carrier to pick up the cans, I hoped Kerri wouldn't be upset that I was giving away some of our remaining food.

While waiting, I got online to check out whether or not this effort was part of a greater plan to help end hunger. I discovered that of the forty thousand or so feeding programs nationwide, most stay away from working on the policy end of the hunger issue and do very little to change the system that creates food insecurity. In reading the work of Joel Berg, the executive director of the New York City Coalition Against Hunger, who also served for eight years under the Clinton administration working at the USDA on several high-profile initiatives to fight hunger, I learned that "trying to end hunger with food drives is like trying to fill the Grand Canyon with a teaspoon." The problem, according to Berg, is that local charities cannot possibly feed the 36.2 million people who need it; that their valiant efforts are only reaching 3.6 percent of those people suffering from food insecurity; and that many of these groups don't focus enough on helping people become self-reliant. At their record-breaking best, these organizations are doing very little to address the overall problem.

Mark Winne, who spent twenty-five years as the executive director of the Hartford Food System in Hartford, Connecticut, explains that food banks and large national feeding organizations generally do not speak up to promote a national conversation about hunger, food insecurity, and poverty because they don't want to alienate the corporate leaders who serve on their boards, who are also influential in government.

Winne's analysis makes sense, but recognition of this alone won't solve the problem. Of course, it doesn't mean that the efforts of food banks and charities are useless—quite the contrary. But it signals that these groups should also push for changes in policy, as well as help their participants become more self-sufficient, as opposed to just handing out food. In fact, these organizations are possibly the ones best equipped to do so. I was pleased to find that our local group does more. The Community Resource Center works to help community members find access to employment, medical treatment, mental health services, affordable child care, and enrollment in the food stamp program, among other services. Self-sufficiency is an integral part of their vision. When I looked out the window again, the bag at the mailbox had disappeared.

Sunday morning, I cooked tofu scramble and hash browns, and we each had three-quarters of a cup of orange juice. The Thrifty Food Plan called for pancakes, but as we were still catching up with our leftovers, we substituted breakfast with a meal option from earlier in the week that our morning rush made difficult. After we enjoyed our carefully planned portion sizes, Kerri got to work on seeing how much money we had left and mapping out our menu for the week.

Remembering my grocery store revelations, I did a survey of the contents of our fridge, freezer, and cupboards to come up with a detailed inventory of what we had left. Items such as a half bulb of garlic, two slices of bread, and a third of a bag of lima beans went into our calculations. With only a week left, $27.75 to spend on food, and a pantry nearing a historic low, we would have to do our best to follow the Thrifty Food Plan while enduring the pressures of supermarket prices that seemed at odds with our budget. While standing in the kitchen and looking at the list of ingredients we needed, and the amount of money we had left, we wondered why certain items were more expensive than others. Why did one store charge two dollars more for an item than the store across the street? With fuel prices coming down from record highs, why had food costs not adjusted six months later? Was the size of this box of cereal actually shrinking?

Now, we aren't economists. We aren't grocery store executives. We don't process or manufacture food, nor do we transport it. And we definitely don't grow it to sell it. Our role in the food production machine is confined to that of the consumer; we are at the end of the line. We shop, we cook, and we eat—which I assume makes us a lot like everyone else. We aren't really sure why the cost of produce goes up or down, and we have little insight into why raw ingredients like corn, soy, and wheat are more expensive than ever. Driving from store to store to get the best deal on beans was not only time-consuming, but an extra hassle that most people wouldn't endure. But after doing some basic research, we learned that there are a number of factors that determine why particular food items cost what they do, some of which we knew of, but many of which we are still learning about. There was one thing we knew for sure: We needed healthy, affordable food.

An article by Mike Hughlett in the *Chicago Tribune* that came out the day after Christmas explained why it would be a while until consumers felt some relief at the supermarket, even though commodity prices had fallen dramatically since summer. Essentially, the article stated that it would take months for the savings in decreased fuel costs to work their way through the intestines of the American food machine. While companies had already enjoyed the benefits of cheaper inputs, most of us were still eating their products, and paying through the teeth for them. The plain economic logic—there was no incentive to cut prices unless the competition started doing so—made sense from a business perspective. But meanwhile, the consumers who bore the burden of rising prices to cover the increase in fuel costs were now being exploited to expand the profit margin. This, of course, was not the only way that food companies were making more money.

Kerri's grandfather, who spent his career in the corporate office of a grocery retailer, said that someone should do an exposé on the shrinking size of food products. While this may not come as a surprise to many people, companies have continued to charge the same amount for things like mayonnaise, even though they have shrunk the size of the jar. The volume has changed, but the cost is the same. From yogurt and cereal to coffee and peanut butter, short-sizing (as it's called in the industry) is an all-too-common way to pass off cost increases to customers. And it is being done all over the store. In order to avoid this scheme, we did what cost-cutting shoppers have been doing since the modern grocery store started: We shopped around and looked for the best price per ounce on nearly everything, which often meant buying in bulk, or at least buying a larger container of the product. However, the Thrifty Food Plan made this practical approach extremely difficult, as we didn't have enough money to get the best deals.

In addition, we learned that while we had the luxury to shop around in our community, we were actually already paying less than what low-income Americans are offered at the stores in their neighborhoods. DeNeen Brown, a writer for *The Washington Post*, detailed some of this phenomenon in an article titled, "Poor? Pay Up." She found that the smaller corner markets serving low-income communities do not have the purchasing power to get the low wholesale cost that the larger suburban markets do, and other costs, such as housing, going to the Laundromat, and fees at check-cashing bureaus, accompanied by lower pay, make being poor in urban areas quite expensive.

Of course, what is not included in DeNeen's calculations is the time spent waiting for public transportation, waiting in line at the medical clinic, the risk and worry involved with living in an area that has a higher crime rate, as well as the missed educational opportunities that abound in wealthier suburban schools. The stress experienced by individuals living in such conditions takes a serious toll on their heath, and with a lack of affordable healthy food, as well as concerns that are far more pressing than getting into a spin class after work, it becomes easier to understand why people like us, in the privileged class, have little real understanding as to why programs like food stamps and other initiatives to address poverty are so essential.

If we were struggling to follow the Thrifty Food Plan in our suburban upper-middle-class community, where the farmers market is the place to be on Sundays, and the gym is always busy, our experiment was clearly an inaccurate way to truly understand what it's like to have to eat on food stamps. Though we did not start our experiments in low-cost eating with these more global implications in mind, the reality check it provided as we approached our last week on the Thrifty Food Plan had humbled us further, and we longed to have this conversation with others. So while food prices started to come down in 2009, the challenges facing Americans living in poverty continued to grow, and our experiment continued to change us.

Macaronipalooza: A Pasta Extravaganza

Kerri

Ordinarily, I feel that I know my way around the kitchen, and I pride myself on my cooking ability. However, there were times during this project that I found myself making stupid rookie mistakes. Recipes we made the last week called for a couple different varieties of pasta. During one shopping trip, Christopher and I decided to save some money by purchasing a large inexpensive bag of macaroni, which was the best deal, instead of a smaller bag and an additional bag of noodles. I would just substitute macaroni for other pastas in the recipes. When I made the saucy beef noodle casserole one night, I replaced the noodles with the macaroni without considering that they might have a different volume when cooked. It even felt wrong as I scooped out the pasta into the pot.

Halfway through, I took the bag into the room where Christopher was working. I asked him, "Does this look right?" There was nowhere near the amount I needed, and I had used almost half of the large bag. True to his own strict cooking style that never departs from the recipes, Christopher shrugged and said, "What did the recipe say?" When I told him how much, he responded, "If it says six and a half, that is what you should do."

Back in the kitchen, I put the pot back on the stove and continued to measure until I had almost emptied the whole bag. As it cooked, I kicked myself. Lesson learned: Macaroni doubles in size. By the time it was ready, there was more than twice the amount that I would need for the casserole. I set aside the excess, threw the ingredients for the casserole into the baking dish, and put it in the oven. It was clear that we'd be eating quite a bit of macaroni during our last week. I checked the cupboard to see if we had what we needed for the chili, which was served over it, then pulled out some containers to store it.

Despite the macaroni mishap and the larger-than-usual amount of pasta we ate that week, things were going well. With only a few weeks left of school, we were wrapping up projects and grading. We were spending more time at school, and less time with each other. One evening, when we both got home around seven p.m., neither of us wanted to cook. We had leftovers in the fridge—namely, dishes that contained macaroni—in addition to another large bowl of the pasta that wasn't yet mixed into anything. We tossed around dinner ideas, but nothing we had sounded appealing. Christopher said, "You know why nothing sounds good? It's because what I really want is a Rico's burrito." I had been thinking the same thing.

While in the dollar-diet project that would have been out of the question, this time there didn't seem to be a reason that we couldn't use some of our supplemental funds for eating out. We started discussing whether or not we could afford it. I sat down to do the math. With only seven days left and the amount of leftovers and pasta in our fridge, we might be able to make it, but it would be close; we'd be eating nothing but macaroni for the rest of the week. I whined that I didn't want to continue eating as much pasta as we had been. I was sick of it, and I told him that I felt as if I was gaining weight. To illustrate my point, I pulled my shirt up and grabbed a roll to show him. According to the scale, I hadn't actually put on any extra pounds, but I felt as if I had, and the vast quantities of carb-loaded pasta were the perfect item to blame. It took me back to my first year of college, when my roommate (who had little room to speak) felt he needed to point out that I was making my way toward the "freshman fifteen." Pasta is cheap, and an easy way to feed large groups of people. It comes as no surprise that it's a common item in dining halls and the apartments of college students.

But now I was looking for sympathy about my perceived weight gain. Instead, Christopher laughed at me and said, "Why don't you write about it?" Since we had begun chronicling our adventures in eating, every concern, complaint, or success was an occasion to write. Needless to say, this suggestion didn't go over well with me. I gave him a dirty look and grabbed the calculator again to find out if we could pull it off. I don't know why I believed that a burrito would be healthier than the pasta, but I wanted one anyway.

We pondered the money we had left, and our cupboard inventory list. Could we stretch our food budget by eating whatever was cheap or should we stick to the original goal of eating what the meal plan asked us to until we ran out of money and food? In the end, we couldn't find a way to justify spending the ten dollars it would cost to eat out and decided to do the best we could to eat close to the meal plan menus for the rest of the week. Fortunately, the week before, we'd had a bit of luck that saved us some money.

Usually a trip to our mailbox is followed by a stop at our recycle bin to throw out the flyers and ads from companies we haven't yet called to get off their junk mail lists. During our third week, I walked down the driveway, expecting much of the same. When I opened the mailbox, I found the usual: bills and junk. Then a bright red card, slightly larger than a postcard, caught my eye. I unfolded it and found our golden ticket. It was an advertisement for the grand opening of a store in our area. It was the same chain, Smart and Final, where we bought most of our bulk items during our first project, but now they were opening a second location about a mile from where the old store had been. Geared toward typical shoppers rather than bulk buyers, this store promised the same low prices with smaller, more convenient sizes. The prices seemed unbelievably low, such as four avocados for a dollar. It seemed too good to be true. I skipped into the house to share the serendipitous event with Christopher.

On the day of the grand opening, Christopher put the announcement in my purse so I wouldn't forget to stop on my way home. As usual, my mind was racing with the million things that needed to be taken care of at school, but that morning I felt like I needed an energy boost to get through all of them. As coffee wasn't a part of our thrifty budget, I plugged in Bon Jovi and turned up the volume. This was a ritual that started during our dollar project. One day when I was exhausted, I chose Bon Jovi for the music to play as the students came in. I sang along loudly as they filed in. Some looked at me as if I was crazy, others began to sing along. A tradition was born. We referred to these mornings as "Bon Jovi days," and it wasn't long before my entire first period class could sing along. Of course, their favorite song was "Livin' on a Prayer," which is about a young couple trying to make ends meet. My undying love for Jon Bon Jovi became a running joke, and students would find ways to work his pictures into presentations, hoping to score some points with me. But this actually served its purpose to help me feel more energized.

After work, as I was chasing the last few debaters out of my classroom and packing up to leave, I found the flyer and remembered my mission. The store is only a few minutes from my school, and on the way home. The shopping center is typically empty, but I had to wait through two green lights before I was able to turn into the parking lot, and there was a line of cars stacking up behind me. Shopping carts and bargain hunters complicated the search for a parking spot, but I waited patiently as a car packed full of white-haired ladies slowly backed out, and I was able to pull in. Encinitas is a fairly affluent area, and I wondered if the crowds were proof that there are hidden poor in every area, or if even the middle- and upper-middle-class shoppers were feeling the pinch of the economy.

True to the promises, the prices were some of the best I had seen, although some of the produce left something to be desired. The four-for-$1 avocados all could have fit easily into one of my hands. Still, there were bargains to be found, and I, as well as half the town, was anxious to get my share. The scene inside was not much different from the parking lot. Crowds of people gathered around the islands of produce with large shopping carts, filling them up with low-priced fruits and vegetables. I had to wait to use a scale to weigh my broccoli as people checked to make sure they were getting no more than the maximum limit for the deals.

Reading the signs, I wondered if they weren't a bit misleading. It seemed as if it would be easy for people to misread the signs and buy more than they needed. For example, the white onions were labeled as ten pounds for one dollar. I started to load my bag when I noticed that underneath the price in smaller print, it said "with Smart Advantage card and designated quantities." It sounded as if it was necessary to buy ten pounds in order to get the deal. I have a college degree—I should have been able to figure this out. But as I was filling a bag full of more onions than we could use in three weeks and trying to remember if I still had my onion soup recipe, I realized that I probably didn't have to buy the full ten pounds. I asked a clerk to clarify. He joked that I would actually have to buy twenty pounds, before telling me that I could buy any amount for ten cents per pound. Relieved, I put over half of the onions back. I smiled to myself as I pushed my cart on and overheard two women by the carrots asking each other the same question.

Eventually I navigated through the masses to the checkout counter. Miraculously, I found a short line. Once I had loaded my goods onto the belt, I looked at the onions; I still had too many. I took three more out of the bag and ran them back to the produce department. I was proud of myself. I was hungry when I got to the store, but I didn't wander or stray too far from my list. My only splurge was bananas. At the end of the trip, I had come home with two pounds of broccoli, four pounds of bananas, three pounds of white onions, one pound of Roma tomatoes, three pounds of carrots, and two heads of lettuce, one romaine and one green leaf, and I only spent $5.07. We celebrated by having a salad with lettuce, tomato, and carrots with our dinner, instead of the suggested half-cup of lettuce and dressing.

I figured that this produce would help to carry us to the end of our project. With only about twenty dollars left and food remaining in the pantry, it seemed as if we could make it through with no problem. But, as I reached for an onion to make another dish of the saucy beef noodles, one of the few dishes that we both enjoyed, I found that all of the remaining onions had mold growing on them. Having gotten over some of my squeamishness about spoiled food during our dollar project, I pulled a knife out of the block and began cutting the bad spots away, throwing them into the tray for the compost bin. I put the rest of the onions in a container for the fridge, hoping to preserve them a little longer.

MOTHER'S DAY FELL on the coming Sunday. Lynda, Christopher's mom, wanted us to meet her for coffee that morning, along with Christopher's sister. Secretly concerned about being able to afford treating her to coffee, I tried to make excuses and convince her that maybe we could go out the following week. But she was persistent, and I can't say that it wasn't appealing to get out of the house. Just as we had in September, we were spending quite a bit of time alone at home that month. I did want to go, but the problem was that I had to tell her, "Lynda, we'd love to take you out for coffee, but we can't afford to right now." Part of Christopher's stubbornness comes from his mother, and on Mother's Day, we found ourselves at a local coffee shop. Lynda treated me to coffee, and Christopher to hot chocolate. She was good-natured and knew we were trying to be "Thrifty," but she couldn't resist teasing us about trying to dodge her. When she and I went up to the counter to order, she told the cashier, "It's Mother's Day and *I'm* taking out my kids." The girl behind the counter smiled. I wanted to explain to her that it was just that we couldn't afford it right then, and that if we had waited a week, it would have been okay. Instead, I thanked her for the coffee and sat down. Typical of Lynda, she was concerned about our health, but was glad to see that we were doing just fine.

But that Mother's Day was not our best in terms of health choices. Our friend Stacy, who had brought us donuts from Las Vegas, also likes to bake. When Stacy, who is also vegan, bakes, we benefit from it. Every once in a while, we get a phone call from her or her husband to find out if they can stop by to drop off treats. On that day, it was an assortment of homemade vegan cookies, donuts, and cupcakes. We sampled one of everything throughout the course of the day. They were delicious, but topped off with fried zucchini and mashed potatoes for dinner, it was a bad day for nutrition.

In general, we were still attempting to prepare as many of the meals from the two-week plan as we could, but to make the money last, we were using up all of our leftover ingredients to make as many of the dishes as possible. This led to repeats and reheats of the same meals, and some odd dinner combinations.

Our last shopping trip was carefully planned out. We spent time again looking over the menus and pantry shelves, and calculated and recalculated how much we had left to spend. One of the menu items that we had not yet tried was the recipe for baked chicken nuggets. Like the crispy chicken that we had enjoyed, it was chicken coated in cornflakes. We were out of cornflakes, so in order to make the meal, we would need to get some, as well as a chicken substitute. At the store, after several minutes comparing prices, we found that it was less expensive to get the processed vegetarian chicken nuggets than to purchase the items needed to make our own. We didn't take the time to consider the health benefits of making our own nuggets versus eating prepackaged ones. Instead, we noted how much easier it would be to throw these into the microwave or oven, not to mention that it saved us a few extra cents. At the register, we came within a couple of dollars of our limit for the month. We considered buying a pack of gum or running back for an extra can of tomato sauce to make it an even total, but decided against it. That turned out to be a good decision.

With only a few days left on the Thrifty Food Plan, I came home from work to find Christopher in a bad mood. He hadn't slept well the night before, and then had had a rough day at work. He was frustrated and upset by a situation that had been escalating for a few weeks. Christopher's social justice students were trying to complete their projects and felt that their efforts were being unfairly stalled or halted by another teacher. Christopher was doing everything he could, but ultimately felt alone in his efforts to help them. We talked through it for a while, but it did little to alleviate his stress. I told him to go take a nap while I made dinner; it might help if he was rested. Then I had an idea. The night before we started this project, we had purchased a chocolate bar, with the intentions of eating it that night. However, we'd had a big dinner, and the chocolate bar had been put in the fridge until the end of the month. I knew we had a couple dollars left. I walked into the living room, where he was lying on the couch.

I rubbed his temples and said, "If you want, we can have that chocolate bar for dessert." Given Christopher's love for anything chocolate, I thought he might appreciate the treat.

He looked up at me sheepishly and admitted, "I ate that weeks ago."

"What? Are you serious?"

While I could forgive him for the cookies, I was shocked that he would sneak the chocolate bar behind my back and never tell me, especially since he had the perfect opportunity when we were confessing our earlier indiscretions. On top of that, we had to add in another $2.55, which took us within a few cents of our total, and I didn't even get one piece.

"I can't believe you'd do that. We have to count that now, and you didn't share," I said as I turned to stomp out of the room.

"Sorry," he said, smiling now, "I just couldn't resist."

"Well, I hope you feel good about yourself!" I shouted from the kitchen as I pulled out dishes to start on dinner. "I wouldn't have done that to you."

With four days left on our Thrifty Food Plan, we found ourselves in a situation not much different from the one before we started our dollar project. We had no money left to spend, so a trip to the store was out of the question. We had only lemonade, popcorn, spaghetti, one can of kidney beans, flour, and hamburger buns left. There were a few remaining chicken nuggets and a small container of leftovers. The other food in the house was the beans and cornmeal in bulk that were left over from September. However, we hadn't charged ourselves for those during our thrifty diet, so we couldn't eat them.

When we started this project, we did not outline rules as strict as we had with the dollar-diet project. We didn't plan to survive for three days on plain noodles, kidney beans, and popcorn; we had done that in September. We had talked before about what we would do at this point, but never come to an agreement.

Christopher argued that since our goal was to see how far we could make our money go, we should stop once we ran out, something he had been asserting since the beginning of the project. My argument was that people in this situation do not have the opportunity to "stop" when they run out, as people receiving SNAP benefits often run out before the month is over. Although our experience was nothing like that of people with limited means, we were trying to gain some perspective about the issue, and we learned firsthand that the money really does run out, even with careful planning. Because of our tight budget, we were no longer following the menu recommendations as closely as we had originally, and due to the leftovers and odd combinations, we were certain that we weren't eating according to the food pyramid.

We came to a compromise: We would finish that day, a Thursday, and go through lunch the following day. We would eat the leftovers for dinner that night, and the remainder would go into my lunch for Friday. Christopher would take the last few chicken nuggets. After that, we would stop. While I was a little disappointed that we didn't make it all the way through, I was glad to be finished.

Peanut Butter Cheesecake

Christopher

The week following the conclusion of living on the Thrifty Food Plan was a whirlwind. The pressure of ending the school year continued to wind us up pretty tightly, but Kerri's birthday was only a few days away, which gave us something to look forward to. Moving away from the USDA's menu gave us both a much-needed sense of relief. We now had one less thing to worry about and could more intensely focus on work. After having been restricted to a limited budget and a plan that relied heavily on white rice, white bread, white flour, and other processed foods like cornflakes and pasta, we were overjoyed to go our own way. Once again we could enjoy foods that we had seen little of while following the plan: burritos from Rico's and chocolate soy milk shakes from Nature's Express (our vegan fast-food drive-through). Our lunches would be free from the banality of milky potato soup, and our dinners filling enough without some type of cabbage worked in.

However, the transition away from the plan was anything but smooth. The excitement over our culinary autonomy blinded us, and we failed to plan our meals adequately. We reverted back to the fly-by-the-seat-of-our-pants dining, which was not only more expensive than a dutifully planned menu, but nutritionally scattered, as well. There were some good elements of our new habits that persisted in the days following the plan. I continued to drink a cup of orange juice every morning, and a cup of soymilk with dinner each night. I even continued to measure my cereal out in the morning, and made sure to pack our lunches with some type of protein source and a fruit or vegetable. There were a couple of nights that week when I recommended one of the meal options that I enjoyed from the menu, like the turkey chili over macaroni, the crispy chicken, or the saucy beef pasta, but Kerri wasn't interested; the revulsion was written in her face.

We generally don't eat some type of meat substitute or dairy several times a day, and the Thrifty Food Plan makes those options some of the most visited foods on the menu. While I rather enjoy the taste of meaty options—not unusual for a vegan—Kerri doesn't get as excited about them as I do, and she was longing for something different. She yearned for a big salad, beans and rice, and other simple foods. This is part of what made it so hard for her to follow the Thrifty Food Plan, even with the alterations we made as we worked our way through the month. Although her personal tastes were far from accommodated, this distaste for the foods in the plan wasn't the only challenge we faced with what the USDA has set out as a guide for low-income families.

We recognize that the task undertaken by the USDA of planning a single menu to help guide the general public on how to eat is beyond difficult, especially when everyone's lives, tastes, family sizes, cultural values, income levels, and nutritional needs are incredibly diverse. But when considering how to build a menu for people to use while planning meals, the USDA needs to reconsider many of its assumptions. For example, it assumes that people on the plan are receiving the average SNAP benefit, that they have a family of four, and that they are able to spend up to 30 percent of their income in addition to using food stamps. Kerri and I, as working adults without children who earn a middle-class income and have debt levels close to the national average, don't represent that target family.

Without a traditional culinary heritage per se, we are pretty average. We like good-tasting, filling food with prep time that fits within our schedules. We like to feel that our meals are healthy, and we don't mind spending time to plan weekly menus. We are vegan, so we don't eat animal products; and we also try not to buy, for instance, produce picked by migrant workers where the labor practices are questionable.

That being said, we let go of most of our political identity to try to follow this plan. We only bought organic when it was the same price, nothing we bought for the plan was local or fair trade, and we shopped mostly at traditional chain supermarkets. Replacing animal protein with comparable plant-based sources wasn't a problem.

Our main challenges stemmed from the fact that the plan is designed for four people, and that the prep time for many of the meals was beyond what we could manage with full-time jobs. In addition, the nutritional value of the meals seemed lacking, and when we looked up the nutritional facts about these foods, we found that we were correct. One example would be the plan's use of orange juice for a serving of fruit, instead of just telling people to eat an orange, which has more vitamins and nutrients. While the foods suggested in the Thrifty Food Plan may fall within the traditional food pyramid, the focus on eating foods made from white flour, meat, and dairy, and only using vegetables and fruits as supplemental (such as a piece of fruit for a snack) flies in the face of what we know about eating. Our diets should be mostly made up of fruits, vegetables, and whole grains, of which there were little in this plan. There were many times when purchasing a larger size in order to get the best value was impossible, given the amount of money we had to shop with. These concerns matter even more because we are privileged in that we have time to spend hours planning and shopping around for bargains. We take eating seriously, we have money, we have transportation—and still it was a struggle to follow the Thrifty Food Plan.

At its core, this program is supposed to be designed so that those receiving the maximum food stamp allotment can feed their families a nutritionally balanced menu, based on the food pyramid. As our budget for this project was based on the average benefit distribut-ed to SNAP recipients, it was almost a given that we would run out of money, since most people on SNAP do. This is why we also supplemented the benefits with the average income that people liv-ing on food stamps are expected to contribute. The average amount of SNAP benefits has typically been close to three dollars a day per person, but it is different for each individual based on a variety of factors, including how many people live in your household. The maximum allotment, which is what the plan is based on, is at least $2.50 more per person, per day. If it's just one person, the maximum amount is more than double the average. Instead of around three dollars, the recipient is given $6.67 per day, which is close to the average spent by most people in the United States each day on food. If someone is actually getting the maximum allotment, then this plan is more than reasonable, but to design a plan that is only af-fordable to those people receiving the maximum benefit makes little sense. The plan should be designed for the average recipient, there-fore making it useful to the largest number of people possible.

Obviously, a big challenge was that the plan is designed for a fam-ily of four. This was clear, as the quantity of leftovers in our fridge forced us to move menu options around, which had the added effect of altering the nutritional balance of the menu overall.

Yet the average family on food stamps with children only has 3.3 people, and the average household size receiving these benefits overall is 2.3 people. While some people may not have children, they may have someone who is disabled, or an elderly person living with them. Thus, the menu for a family of four is too big to begin with. This means that the people the plan was actually created for, much like us, will have to modify it in order accommodate a differ-ence between SNAP benefits and the actual cost of the Thrifty Food Plan, as well as adjust it for a smaller family size. The in-store reality of a problem like this is that for those trying to follow the plan, or use it as a guide, foods like cereal, loaves of bread, and juice do not come in very many sizes, which forces people to buy the smaller size, thereby getting less for their money. The plan as it stands now doesn't have the largest number of people in mind; it is built for a family of four receiving the maximum allotment, so a family of, say, five would really have trouble making do with SNAP.

These built-in assumptions about the amount of assistance, and the family size of the households receiving that assistance, do not match reality. The USDA knows that the cost of the plan doesn't match up with the average SNAP benefit, as their own documentation shows. In April 2009, a family of two between the ages of nineteen and fifty years old could expect to pay $350 to eat on the Thrifty Food Plan, according to the USDA. The USDA documents the cost of the plan monthly in order to record how food prices shift over time. With our average allotment on SNAP, plus the supplemental income, our total budget for both of us was $249.60. This shortfall doesn't make sense. At the cost of food when we did this, we were one hundred dollars short. However, if we were receiving the maximum benefit for two people, we would have had just enough to make it work.

Beyond these structural problems with the plan, we found that as people with full-time jobs, we didn't have the time to prepare most of the lunches without serious changes to the meal (for instance, prepackaged frozen burgers instead of ground meat), or making the lunch meal the night before at the same time that we made dinner. The rice cereal listed for breakfast took twenty-five minutes to cook, and this extra time in the morning made me late for work. The amount of preparation and cooking time required for dinners was more than we typically had the patience for, and in these instances we were thankful when we had leftovers. While some of the dinners, like the stir-fry, take as little as twenty-five minutes from start to finish, most take about an hour (give or take), with some, like the chili, taking closer to two hours. Of course, when you are making a new meal for the first time it takes a little longer. We weren't in the habit of making things like the (unpalatable) turkey-cabbage casserole, and pulling such dishes together took a little bit longer than the times listed on the recipes.

There were many nights when eating a burrito from our local

taco shop would have been far less stressful, and a couple of times we considered it, but with the limited budget, we could not afford the four-dollar luxury. That being said, if the meals had tasted better, or appealed to us, we would have been less frustrated when preparing them. After working a ten-hour day, it's disheartening to spend valuable time preparing a meal that doesn't sound that appetizing to begin with. But as this is solely an issue of personal taste, we would simply like to recommend that the plan become more diverse in its offerings.

The plan is also inconsistent with the options listed for snacks. Some days it lists French fries or chocolate pudding (far from healthy), and on other days it suggests orange juice. On one day, there is no snack at all. As a side note, as mentioned earlier, the plan also assumes that you already have spices like garlic powder, chili powder, dried parsley flakes, dried oregano, dry mustard, and paprika. Luckily we had them, but the spices themselves are not included on the USDA shopping list, and since spices are often expensive, it would be hard to rationalize a three-dollar container of dry mustard that would be used infrequently, versus a complete frozen dinner or loaf of bread for the same price. In addition, the plan also assumed that we had the equipment to make the food they suggested: pots, pans, mixing bowls, and baking dishes.

In comparison to the dollar-diet experiment, the Thrifty Food Plan allowed us more flexibility in our food planning, more nutritionally balanced meals, and adequate serving sizes. It also allowed us more diversity in menu options, and it took less of a toll on our personal health. Kerri and I both maintained our weight, although we didn't do any strenuous exercise, and the only times we felt pangs of hunger were when we made a mistake in our planning. Our lack of time made it hard to stay active, and hard to plan.

As a guide for those with little money to spend on food, the Thrifty Food Plan needs a serious overhaul. Having had the experience with the dollar diet, we knew the benefit of planning meals around central ingredients like beans and rice, potatoes, and tomato sauce. We knew that it was better to go shopping for fewer processed food products and more raw ingredients, and to judge costs on the price per ounce. And we understood the necessity of planning for leftovers as a way to reduce waste, save time, and control portion sizes. While each experiment had its benefits and challenges, after finishing each one, we felt fortunate that we could take what we learned and apply those lessons to our lives.

The one factor that was missing from both projects was that we didn't feel particularly healthy during either one. We had managed to survive while spending far less than we had in the past, and far less than the average American spends on food each day. But is survival the objective, or do we also want people to thrive?

The amount of fresh produce in each plan wasn't nearly enough for our ideal diet. We were left wanting more, and in our community, "more" is everywhere. We now understand why people in low-income areas are more likely to stop at a fast-food restaurant than go home and cook up, say, the baked cod with cheese and scalloped potatoes that the Thrifty Food Plan suggests. Fast food is convenient, satisfying, and appears to be cheap, especially if one eats from the dollar menu. This is also why many of the poorest among us suffer from obesity and other health problems.

However, our area is far different from the one where those most underserved by the food stamp program live. While fast-food options exist in our community, we rarely visit them. You would have to make an effort to go to one, and if you are going out, it makes more sense to patronize one of the local restaurants or taco shops instead. In our coastal community, things are pretty spread out; you need a car to get from residential areas to places to shop or to access other community services. There are few people walking around outside, even in the busiest sections of town. Most of the people who live here are white, and when it comes to income level, as of 2007, the median household income was above $90,000. There are about 60,000 people living in an area that stretches over roughly twenty square miles, with sandy beaches, coastal shopping districts, and high-performing schools. The median cost of a rented house at the time of this writing is $1,700 a month.

By contrast, in City Heights, the region of San Diego that we discovered had the lowest food stamp participation in the nation, there were people everywhere. Many shops in City Heights are easily accessible without a personal vehicle, the population is predominantly Hispanic, and the median household income is close to $30,000. In City Heights, there are 80,000 people crammed into an area that is three square miles, with mostly family-run markets and bodegas, where 40 percent of adults have less than a twelfth-grade education, and the median cost of a rental, either a house or an apartment, is under $600 a month.

While the residents of Encinitas have several parks, beaches, and fitness centers, which support a greater level of health, those living in City Heights are far younger overall, and have the same hospitalization rate for coronary heart disease as the rest of the entire county. This area also has the highest hospitalization rate for asthma in the county, and it's more than double the rate of our area. Since City Heights is the densest neighborhood in San Diego, houses are often infested with cockroaches and mold, which, beyond being unsanitary, contribute to children suffering from acute symptoms.

When we visited City Heights, we noticed that liquor stores had prime real estate, while in our community one is more likely to see wine merchants tucked in between Italian restaurants and upscale boutiques. These differences between our area and City Heights heightened our understanding about the level of privilege that we are accustomed to, and helped us further understand that while we had merely limited the amount of money we spent on food, there were a number of interconnected factors that determine a person's ability to maintain a healthy lifestyle. Eating well is actually encouraged in our area through several large supermarkets, natural food stores, healthy dining options, open spaces, and recreational activities; the same cannot be said for places like City Heights, where far more people reside within far less space.

However, beyond their differences, both areas of San Diego are vibrant places where people live and work, doing their best to build better lives for themselves and their communities. People in both areas deserve to have the opportunity to choose healthy options at affordable prices, but unfortunately this is not the case, and for those receiving SNAP benefits, it is even more challenging. It's definitely not as easy as stopping by the Whole Foods on the way home from work to pick up some arugula for a salad. And while educational efforts to help people understand healthy eating patterns are important, they are useless unless such foods are readily available and priced within their budget. People tend to know which foods are healthy. They don't need a class; they need a paycheck.

With our experience eating on the Thrifty Food Plan behind us, we continued to wonder what it truly costs for people to eat a healthful diet. We had lived more or less in line with the food pyramid for just over four dollars a day, but with the average American spending seven dollars a day on food, why were so many people suffering from diet-related health problems like obesity and heart disease? Was it what they were eating? How was it possible that in the richest nation on Earth, many people were still suffering from food insecurity, while struggling with being overweight? Did it really cost more to eat well? Were people in our country, rich and poor alike, just eating too much? These questions lingered as the week passed and Kerri's birthday approached.

AT OUR HOUSE, we treat birthdays like international holidays. We go all out. My birthdays are usually destination birthdays, and when Kerri's come around, I try to go beyond her expectations. This year I was in luck, as her sister had devised a plan to surprise Kerri by getting her family down to our house for a few days, for her thirtieth. Her family doesn't travel much, and as they live at the other end of the state, about six hundred miles away, this was special. Her birthday fell on a Friday, and that night we went to Hollywood to be part of the studio audience for one of our favorite shows, then ate dinner afterward at a restaurant in West Hollywood called Real Food Daily. When we are in this area, and can afford it, we visit one of their two locations; it's a luxury saved for special occasions.

Beyond ballpark fare at a Padres game we'd attended, this was our first meal out in over a month, and it was difficult to decide what to have. We started with the Better Than Cheddar Nachos: tortilla chips topped with melted cashew cheese, black beans, pico de gallo, guacamole, and tofu sour cream. The mountainous plate lasted maybe five minutes. Next, Kerri and I shared the special salad, which included roasted golden beets, sweet peas, soft avocado with romaine lettuce, and a designer dressing. For our entrees, I had the enchiladas stuffed with sautéed and roasted mushrooms, red bell peppers, and other veggies, topped with pico de gallo, and a side of black beans and Spanish rice. Kerri had a Caesar wrap: blackened tempeh, avocado, capers, romaine hearts, and Caesar dressing in a spinach tortilla, accompanied by a side of mashed potatoes topped with mushroom gravy. For dessert, I ordered a "Fauxstess" chocolate cupcake, while Kerri enjoyed espresso. I knew that dinner would be pricey, and as Kerri's family had gone to great expense to visit, I felt it was only appropriate for me to take care of the bill. When the server brought over the little black folder I was stunned: $125 for the four of us. Now, for the celebrities who live in the area, this is probably a steal, but for a schoolteacher who had just spent about that much to feed himself for an entire month, this was beyond comprehension. I thought of those who would never be able to afford this meal. I did some quick rationalizing: It's her birthday. We're in Hollywood. Her family is here. This is a special occasion. I pulled out my wallet and anxiously withdrew my debit card.

The next day we took her family to the beach, and for the first time in over a month, we did not have to vigilantly watch our intake of snacks. I tried to resist the herb and garlic crackers dipped in garlic hummus while we relaxed on the shore, but after a few minutes, I caved in. Kerri put the cracker in my mouth; as the garlic flavor hit my tongue, I closed my eyes in bliss. With each crunch, a feeling of relief washed over me. The box was empty within an hour.

This revived habit of gratification eating continued a few hours later. A larger group of us would be celebrating Kerri's birthday that night at Sipz. We had not eaten there since the end of the dollar-diet project, and once again, the number of choices was overwhelming. The serving sizes seemed relatively normal this time, whereas the day after we finished eating on a dollar a day, they had seemed enormous. Jovial conversation and laughter carried us through our appetizers and entrees, and as Kerri stepped away to the restroom for a moment, I hopped up and found our friend Sylvia, who owned the restaurant.

"Did it come in?" I asked.

She nodded. "We put it in the freezer when it got here, but we took it out this afternoon so it would be ready by the time you arrived. I can't believe you had it shipped here from Philadelphia. It must be really good."

I asked her to bring it out in about five minutes. Returning to my seat before Kerri came back from the bathroom, Kerri's mother asked, "So did it get here all right?"

I answered that it had, and by the smile on my face, the rest of the table could see that this was going to be special. Kerri returned to the table, and right on cue Sylvia approached with the dinner's finale. We sang "Happy Birthday" as people in the restaurant turned to see who the lucky person was, and Kerri blew out the candle.

"Oh wow. Is this what I think it is?" Kerri asked with a look of disbelief.

A year earlier, Kerri and I were in Philadelphia with my journalism students, and we ate at a place called Gianna's Grille. The restaurant caters to omnivores and vegans alike, but their desserts are completely vegan, and some of the best in the world. We made several visits back to Gianna's over the course of our trip, and my students liked it so much that they had it delivered to the hotel. The desserts are so renowned that you can have them shipped overnight across the country. I had put in the order a couple of weeks earlier, and it had arrived: Death by Chocolate and Peanut Butter Cheesecake. Overnight shipping for a refrigerated dessert across the United States isn't cheap, but my sweet tooth combined with this special occasion made the outlandish and extravagant cheesecake an easy choice. Besides, this was something she would remember for the rest of her life. Sylvia handed Kerri the cake knife and she began serving everyone. Upon the first few bites, looks of utter amazement swept the table. Like flowers finding the sun, the faces of those in our group came to life in a current of sheer ecstasy. Peanut butter frosting drizzled over the Oreo chocolate chunk topping gave way to cool layers of fluffy peanut butter cheesecake filling. I smiled at Kerri, and between bites whispered, "I love you."

Yet, as each decadent forkful passed my lips I could not help but call to mind the situation in City Heights, and the people nationwide who were struggling to find enough to eat. I thought about our experiences with the dollar-diet project and the Thrifty Food Plan. I closed my eyes and reminded myself to be thankful for my life, and remembered the promise I had made to myself to do what I could to help. As a person with privilege, I knew that I had a responsibility to speak up when I could, but I was still struggling with my own food battles. Our experiments had brought to the surface my own struggles to eat reasonably sized portions, and challenged me to adhere to healthier eating patterns. It seemed only appropriate to get my eating habits in order before asking anyone else to do likewise. We finished up our hedonistic dessert and went home, thoroughly sated.

Over the next few days, I reflected on what we needed to do in order to help us further understand our relationship to food. We spent a good amount of time deconstructing our budget, and the SNAP program, but we still didn't feel like we had figured out what it meant to "eat well," or how much we were willing to spend in order to do so. We knew that the dollar diet was too extreme for the long term, and that the Thrifty Food Plan wasn't the right menu for our schedules, tastes, or progressive politics.

So, we started making a plan for our next experiment. I did some research online, picked up some books from health experts, started planning a menu, and thought about what it would take for us to eat "healthy." We wondered how much it would cost to eat well, considering our modest budget, our work schedules, and our need for good-tasting, filling food. This was no easy task. Our local paper was always promoting some type of food as a solution to some type of physical ailment. Supermarket checkout stands were choked with magazine food stories that made healthy eating seem effortless, and even fun. Our experiences in trying to improve the way we ate seemed quite contrary. It took effort to plan menus, and after a long day working with teenagers, cooking was anything but fun. In the same spirit that led us to question the cost dynamic of our grocery shopping, we now faced an additional challenge: to focus on our health as well.

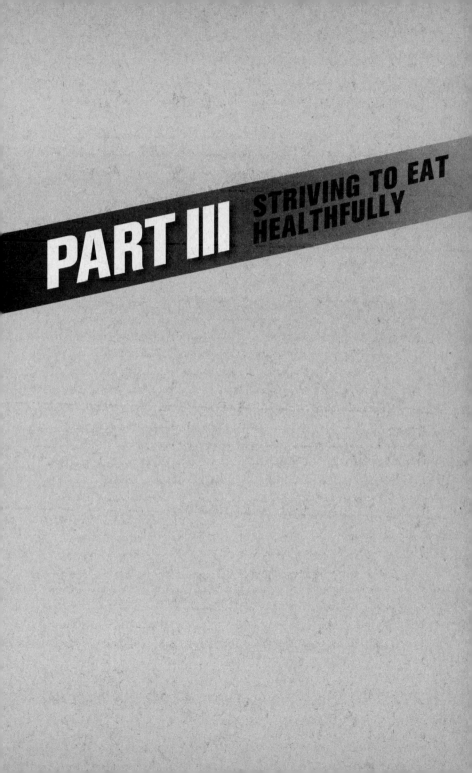

PART III

STRIVING TO EAT HEALTHFULLY

Seventeen Tomato Plants

Kerri

I feel like I need to take more of an active role in fixing our meals."

I was stunned. It was fairly early in the morning, and we were sitting at home in front of our computers when Christopher's comment seemed to come from nowhere. We had previously discussed the fact that I didn't want to be the only one who did the food prep before embarking upon any of our projects, but in the other two cases, I was the one requesting help. This was a first.

Despite the fact that the conversation had started off with a thoughtful offer, it became more intense. This was in part due to my usual knack for choosing the wrong moment to roll out my laundry list of ways I felt that I took on quite a bit of the burden in our experiments. "Great," I said, "because I really feel like I do most of the work."

Oops, that didn't come out quite as I had planned. Christopher stared at me in disbelief. *Had I really just responded to his offer to help by insulting him?*

"I do make you breakfast, and I pack your lunch every day," he offered.

He was right, he did both of these things. This conversation was getting sticky. I needed to dance my way around this, so I took a few breaths before proceeding. It was important for me to let him know how much I appreciated that he did these things for me. I consider the fact that he packs my lunch a bragging point among my girl-friends. It solicits a "You've got a keeper . . . don't let him get away," or "I wish my boyfriend was that thoughtful." I didn't want him to think I took his efforts for granted, but there were times when I felt that mine were.

"I know you do, and I appreciate it more than you know. But I've been planning the meals, making the shopping lists, and all the din-ners. A lot of times when you make dinner, it's just reheating some-thing that took me a long time to make. And while we're doing these projects, a lot of our lunches are leftovers that I packed into contain-ers the night before, so all you're doing is putting them in my lunch bag the next day."

"I was just offering to help," he said, looking hurt.

"I know you were. I didn't mean to rant; I do want your help." We sat at our computers in silence. Neither of us was angry, but I was simultaneously wishing I had found a better time to air my complaints, while also feeling relieved at having shared them. We didn't have time to continue this conversation for now; I had plans to meet Christopher's sister at my school in a few minutes. The school year was over, and she was coming to help me straighten up my classroom for the summer. Heather, like her brother, is incredibly organized, a skill I have yet to master. The last weeks of school, at times, can be more exhausting than the first. While grading stacks of portfolios and conferencing with students to explain why they might have received a B plus instead of an A minus, I also needed to complete my checkout work, turn in grade books for the year, and fulfill a number of other tasks. My classroom began to look like an explosion had gone off, and I needed to clean up so the custodians could get in and do the summer deep-cleaning. I got up from my cluttered desk and kissed Christopher good-bye, leaving him sitting alone at his neatly organized workspace.

When I returned home several hours later, I found Christopher in the same place I had left him: in front of the computer. I walked in with the intention of motivating him to abandon whatever task he was working on so that we could make a grocery list and go shopping before it was too late in the day.

He greeted me, pulled my desk chair next to his, and patted the seat for me to sit down. "I want to show you what I've been working on."

On the screen in front of me was a spreadsheet that outlined two weeks' worth of breakfasts, lunches, and dinners, with optional snacks included. From the looks of it, we would be starting our project by dining on lentil stew, whipped parsnips, baked tofu, and seared kale. There were stars next to three or four of the dinners each week that he planned to make—such as the Jamaican veggie patties—and a couple of empty dinners so that I could pick out what I wanted to make. Next to his computer sat a copy of *Becoming Vegan* by Brenda Davis, R.D., and Vesanto Melina, M.S.R.D., a book that includes a vegan food pyramid and diet plans based on calorie intake needs, as well as several cookbooks and a grocery list based on the menu he had created.

I smiled at him and threw my arms around his neck. "Thanks!"

"That was a lot of work," he remarked. I couldn't help but smile. I knew it was work; that was what I had been trying to tell him for months. I felt as if he now understood why I had been so frustrated.

With the new menu in hand, we set out to take our food experiments in a different direction. This time, with no limited budget, we would eat a healthy diet. A question that we had in the back of our minds, but had never really discussed, was what exactly did "healthy" mean to us?

As Christopher has previously stated, the act of eating is very personal. For example, what constitutes healthy food intake and portion sizes for Christopher, who is almost a foot taller than I am, differs for me. Likewise, what I need differs from the needs of my three-year-old nieces. In addition, people have varying tastes and cultural dietary expectations that determine what they choose to include in a healthy diet.

For us, obviously, we maintained our vegan diets, but worked toward using the wisdom we had gained from the dollar-diet project and the Thrifty Food Plan. The dollar-diet project taught us that we could continue to incorporate whole grains into our diets inexpensively. Furthermore, we learned that we felt better when we monitored our portion sizes. We've both been known to eat beyond feeling full, until we're uncomfortable. Controlling portions would prevent the food coma that can follow such a huge meal. We also tend to eat too much pasta, or too many sweets. From the Thrifty Food Plan, we learned that we wanted to work at having a better balance of foods, such as shown in the food pyramid.

While we didn't outlaw any particular foods, we knew that as much as possible, we wanted to eat whole grains and fresh vegetables; also, we wanted to be able to eat out if we needed to. For example, we were going on a road trip that had been planned far in advance, but we would make healthier choices than we did before our diet adventures. We would eat treats if they were available, but we wouldn't overdo it. Christopher, in particular, is coming to terms with his penchant for sweets. When there are sugary foods in the house, he has to deal with an internal tug-of-war to convince himself not to overindulge. There have been numerous occasions in our life together where we share some cookies, and by the time I go back to the cookie jar a day or two later, they have vanished. Our cookie jar is a relic left over from Christopher's childhood. It is shaped like the stump of a tree, and on top sits a sly raccoon dressed as a thief, slinging a bag over his shoulder as he attempts to break into the cookie safe. This is not unlike Christopher's clandestine nighttime trips to the cookie jar.

As for me, I can control myself when it comes to sweet foods—my weakness is chips and salsa—but my challenge is serving sizes. I don't know where my tendency to overserve myself comes from; perhaps my great-aunt Lily's love of feeding people has rubbed off on me. She is the best cook in the family, and her meals are enough to feed twice as many people as she is serving. I have inherited this need to prepare an abundance of food, despite the fact that there are only two of us eating. When I first met Christopher, he was working on watching his weight. He measured out his breakfast cereal to fit the recommended serving size and ate his dinner off of smaller-sized salad plates to keep from eating too much, a concept I didn't understand. It didn't take long for me to break him of that habit, as I tend to pile our plates high. At times Christopher puts some back, but I usually don't.

Taking our own issues into consideration, we needed to come up with a plan for how to eat. We decided that we would be mindful of what we were spending, but staying under a particular dollar amount was not our goal. We would eat as healthfully as possible, and whenever we could, we would shop in a way that embodied what we believe (i.e., fair trade and organic). Because we were free to spend what we needed to, it would be up to us, not a budget, to keep our portion sizes to reasonable servings. We would eat whole grains and make sure we had several servings of fruits and vegetables each day.

We left the grocery store after our first trip on our new plan having spent $155.38. Our total closely resembled what it had been before we started experimenting. We were surprised that we had spent so much, but the trunk was loaded with a cornucopia of lettuce, carrots, nectarines, blueberries, and strawberries, along with several different grains. When we got home, I set to work putting groceries away while Christopher started dinner: baked tofu with mashed parsnips and a green salad. As we finished eating, he told me that he had dessert planned and took my plate to the sink for me. I was instructed not to look so that I could be surprised. He returned with a small bowl of blueberries and strawberries. The berries had the perfect amount of tartness and were just sweet enough to be a delicious end to our meal. It was nice to have dessert, and a much better choice than the chocolate we usually go for.

It was immediately apparent to us that while food was a large part of it, being healthy came from much more than just what we ate. In terms of healthy living, we had an advantage over many people. As we learned at the Food Justice conference, zip code, stress levels, and physical exercise were key factors in obesity rates. As stated before, we live in an area where we have a plethora of health food stores, farmers markets, and grocery stores. Our stress levels were about to be greatly reduced, since the start of this new project coincided with the end of our school year. This left us enough time on our hands to plan and prepare healthy meals and to get daily exercise. We promised ourselves to go to the gym at least four times a week and to do some type of physical activity for at least thirty minutes every day.

While the prospect of this project was far more appealing than the other two, in some ways planning it was just as difficult. Health isn't something that can be achieved in one month, after which you're set for life; it needs to be maintained. We decided that we didn't want this to be a one-month deal, we wanted to make a permanent lifestyle change that we would continue indefinitely. This month would be a trial run for how we wanted to live our lives. It wasn't a month to work on weight, but to work on feeling healthy, energized, and good about how we were nourishing our bodies. This seemed to clash with the emphasis our culture puts on weight; looking good in our "skinny" jeans is often more important than overall well-being.

During junior high and high school, I watched my parents and parents of friends try different diets. The one that sticks out for me was when my parents made a pot of some kind of soup at the beginning of the week and divided it into serving-size portions to last the week. They would add a variety of vegetables and grains on different days, according to the diet's plan, and that was what they had for dinner each night. (I can't remember what my sisters and I had for dinner, but we only ate the soup once or twice.) While a soup diet may help some to lose some weight, realistically it isn't a permanent change that anyone could make. I don't know if either of my parents lost any weight, but I don't think the soup diet lasted for very long.

It's no surprise that my parents were looking for a quick fix, rather than a lasting change in their lives. Fad diets tend to be short-lived and do little to develop healthy lifestyle choices. Before starting our healthy eating plan, we hit the bookstores in our town to see what we could learn. In the nutrition and diet section, we found a wide variety of books about how to lose weight quickly or without giving up the foods you love, but few and far between were the books that talked about making enduring changes to the way we think about food.

On TV there is a constant barrage of commercials about pills, or more recently, machines that can help people lose weight with no effort. When I worked at the grocery store, I had the opportunity to see the outrageous number of magazines geared toward women and teen girls that had tips for losing weight fast, or the latest abdominal workout that required only a few minutes a day to give you that six-pack stomach. My favorite was a magazine that featured on its cover each week women who had lost inordinate amounts of weight, often holding up a pair of their old pants next to their newly thin body, and the promise that readers could find out how they could do this, too. This magazine featured decadent cakes on the same cover. Men are also subject to magazine and TV images of what the ideal male looks like. There are continuous conflicting messages of "eat" or "look like a supermodel." On several occasions during lunch at school, I have overheard teenage girls talking about not eating something or other because they want to lose weight.

Christopher has struggled with weight issues since childhood, so we'd have to consider that while planning our new healthy eating style. I don't have an issue with my weight, but I fight daily battles with self-image. My logical mind recognizes that I am small (five three) and relatively slim, but I still find myself looking in the mirror and dissecting every part of my body, wondering why my legs are not just a little bit longer and a little bit thinner. Countless times I have turned to Christopher to ask, "Does this make me look fat?" or "Does my butt look big in this?" He usually sighs and says, "Why do you ask me that? You know I think you look fine." I have come to realize, though, that when I feel good, no matter what the scale may say, I feel better about myself. Taking back our health included taking control of what we eat. Instead of being bound by the supermarket, we would need to declare our independence, and one way we planned to do this was to start growing our own food.

I have made several attempts at gardening in the five years

Christopher and I have been together. In the first house we lived in, I attempted to grow tomatoes and bell peppers on our back patio, a venture that went well until we took a weeklong trip and I forgot to ask Christopher's sister, who was staying at our house, to water the plants. When we bought our home, I was excited about the raised flower beds in the backyard. I could picture myself tending to my garden and bringing in the small harvest for our dinners. But the two curious toddlers that we call dogs crushed that fantasy.

In early May 2009, I decided to do my gardening on our front patio, an area that the dogs are never in without supervision. This is when my ideas of growing our own food turned into an obsession. When I was younger, it seemed that the only people I knew who were gardening were "old." My grandparents and my great-aunt Lily were the gardeners in my life, and while I loved getting to eat the results of their hard work, I had no interest in taking it up. If asked where produce comes from, I most likely would have rolled my eyes and said, "The grocery store." My own views on where my veggies came from were probably not too far away from those of my niece Kylie, who, at the age of three, laughed at me when I told her that I eat plants. She was skeptical when I told her that some of her favorite foods, cucumbers and strawberries, were plants and they grew in the ground. But now it seems that everyone I know has at least one or two planters where they are growing tomatoes or beans. I've had several in-depth conversations with a student who spent a weekend building raised beds and learning how to make mulch. Even my mom is growing herbs in the backyard. Earlier this year, gardening got a celebrity endorsement when First Lady Michelle Obama started a garden.

As I began to bring home pots and seeds on a weekly basis, Christopher commented that if he knew how much I was into plants, he would have given me a bag of potting soil for my birthday. And it is true: I do love to watch my vegetables grow. What started as a patio garden expanded with my unstoppable desire to plant every seed I could get my hands on.

When we could afford to have a fence put up to keep the dogs out of the garden, we added a few more raised planters in the back-yard. One evening I was out transplanting kale seedlings into the garden. I had on my ridiculous wide-brimmed gardening hat and sunglasses, and I was singing along to Rilo Kiley blasting from my iPod. I had been trying to figure out what had been eating holes in the leaves, thinking it was the birds who had become frequent visitors to our porch. While transplanting, I discovered several small green worms enjoying my kale. Oblivious to my surroundings, I carefully picked each worm off the plants and placed them on the stone of the planter, while I examined the leaves for more intruders. I have no idea how long I was engrossed with my chore, but when I scooped up the worms to relocate them, I screamed, suddenly realizing that someone was standing next to me. It was Christopher.

"How long have you been there?" I asked.

He laughed. "At least five or six minutes. I thought you knew I was here; I didn't know why you were ignoring me."

I relocated my worms to the other side of the fence and turned back to look at my hard day's work. Christopher appreciates the garden, but he doesn't share the same love for the dirt that I do. There's something to be said for taking a tiny seed and watching it grow into a beautiful bunch of chard or bright red tomatoes. However, one of my weaknesses as a gardener is my unwillingness to thin the sprouts. You need to plant more seeds than will be able to survive, so that you can choose the strongest ones to continue growing and pick the smaller ones away. Once something has sprouted, it makes me sad to remove it. I had one starter pot where I had accidentally planted a Swiss chard and a rainbow cherry tomato together. My intention was to separate them, but by the time I was ready to transplant, they were so intertwined that I couldn't tear them apart. Rather than sacrifice one to save the other, I planted them together and figured the strongest plant would win out in the end. As of this writing, that particular chard plant is the biggest, yet the tomato is still thriving. It's when I share information like this that Christopher smiles at me and says, "That's great, baby. It's getting dark; are you going to stay out here all night?"

The garden would take a while to get going, and despite the fact that we had ample space, it wouldn't serve all of our produce needs. It isn't uncommon for people to suggest to us that if we want inexpensive produce, planting a garden is the way to go, and that anyone can do it regardless of space. While I agree to an extent, gardening is not as cheap as I thought it would be. Once things were up and running, the cost of maintaining a garden became affordable, but as a beginning gardener I made plenty of expensive mistakes. Also, with limited space it's possible to grow some vegetables, but not to meet all of the produce needs of a family.

When I started out, I spent a great deal of time and money at the Armstrong Garden Center in Encinitas. I'm not sure that the employees know me by name, but they certainly know my face. On at least two occasions I've run in after work, only a few minutes before they closed, and told an employee that I knew what I was getting and I'd be quick. I was told not to worry; I should take my time. A woman at the counter told me, "Honey, you're so cute, you just take all the time you need. We know you." That made my day—and they *should* know me. For my birthday, I received eighty dollars' worth of gift certificates to Armstrong, and I used them up in two trips.

If I had to start my garden again, there are things I would do differently. For container gardening, one expensive element was the containers themselves. I had some pots at home, but not enough for what I planned to grow. I should have shopped around to find the lowest prices, but instead I stuck to the store I was familiar with. Furthermore, the cost of organic compost and potting soil added up quickly. It wasn't until I was several months into gardening and putting in the beds in the backyard that I considered looking for places to get free or inexpensive compost. While this should have been common sense, I was doing quite a bit of guesswork and Internet research to learn how to garden, as well as taking a few free classes at gardening centers.

The seeds alone don't cost much, but they did cause me another problem. As a first-time gardener, I had no idea how many of my seeds would sprout and survive. I planted a wide variety of vegetables, but too many of each. It was a little late in the season when I started my seeds, so as of this writing, we are still waiting for many of our plants to produce. Our surplus will be shared with friends and family, and I'll also look for a food bank to donate to. Like a chemist in a laboratory, I am going through the process of trial and error to find the right combinations to get the most from our space. I have six different varieties of tomatoes, with seventeen plants. I also have three varieties of chard with seven plants; three types of kale; and six jalapeños. This is in addition to cucumbers, basil, mint, chives, green beans, bok choy, onions, snap peas, arugula, lettuce, salad greens, and leeks. It's going to take me a season or two to figure out how much we need. My backyard is my laboratory, and although my results are inconclusive as of yet, I will continue to search for a formula to help us eat well.

I ran into a coworker, and she and I got on the subject of gardening. I explained to her that I knew I had overplanted. She told me that one of the joys of gardening is sharing and trading with others. She listed three other coworkers who garden and told me that they swap produce all the time. Then she whipped out a pen and paper and asked for my address. Just knowing that I was willing to share prompted her to stop by my house that afternoon with a bag full of peaches and plums from her yard. I hadn't really considered how fulfilling the sharing would be. Christopher's mom stopped by one day to get some basil from me, and I sent her home with green beans, lemon cucumbers, tomatoes, and figs from an old tree that is in our front yard. She was thrilled with the booty she carted off.

While gardening is one thing that we are doing to help us to live a more healthful lifestyle, obviously it isn't something that everyone can do. My inexperience made the start-up costs a bit expensive. Our house sits on almost a quarter of an acre, and we have the room to grow quite a bit of food. We also live in San Diego, which gives us a longer growing season. A friend told me I could plant almost anything year-round, a hypothesis I can't wait to test. I do think it's possible for most people with a yard to grow some of their produce, but it's misleading to say that this is an easy solution to the cost of food. Growing your own veggies isn't an immediate solution, but it might be helpful in the long run if people have the money and time to invest.

To supplement our garden, we signed up for a local CSA (community-supported agriculture). When we called to find out how to sign up, luckily a spot had just opened; usually there is a waiting list. Our CSA is Be Wise Ranch, a local organic farm approximately thirty minutes from our house. We paid $125, which covered our startup fee and four weeks' worth of produce. Each week we would go to a pickup point, which turned out to be less than a mile from our house, and get a "small" box of produce. The boxes contain whatever is in season, and everything within it is freshly picked. This helps us to eat local, fresh, and organic. Due to the time it took to get signed up and started, we didn't get our first delivery until the end of our second week of our healthy eating plan.

Before that, we had already faced a few challenges. Because we were on summer break, going to the gym was easy. We made it a priority; it was the first thing we did when we got up in the morning. Within a few days, we came to realize the positive changes we were seeing and feeling. But the end of our first week was Father's Day weekend. My dad's side of the family has a tradition of getting together at my grandpa's cabin and spending Father's Day weekend with one another. This year it was particularly important that we go, as my grandfather and one of my cousins both had passed away earlier that year. My family needed to come together for a happier occasion.

This meant a road trip for us. My entire family lives in northern California, so for Christopher and me, it is a ten-hour car ride. We left much later than we intended to because we hit the gym before beginning our trip, and we packed a lunch to take with us, so that we didn't have to stop and eat out. Food on the road turned out not to be our biggest challenge. It was easy to drive by the fast-food chains at the freeway off-ramps when our mini ice chest was filled with sandwiches, strawberries, and almonds. However, when we got to my grandpa's cabin in the woods, it was harder to control what we ate.

The laughter of my large family filled the deck of the cabin that my grandfather built. Wading through the hellos and hugs, we passed by two picnic tables covered with an array of snacks. My family members walked by the tables and filled their plates with the chips, dip, and treats that had been laid out. It's hard to resist the crunch of potato chips coming through in surround-sound while everyone else is enjoying them. The sound seemed to increase the pressure to eat the nutrition-deficient snacks. To fight off the urge to dig in, I filled a plate with veggies for Christopher and me to share. They had the same satisfying crunch, but with less salt. We did well throughout the day, sticking to veggies and the food that we brought. But when the cupcakes came out, all bets were off.

My sister Kimberly is famous among my family and friends for the desserts she makes and decorates. Not only does she make things for the whole family, she also takes the extra time to make a batch of vegan treats so that Christopher and I aren't left out. Twelve gorgeous vegan cupcakes on their own separate tray awaited us.

While the concept of "vegan" is foreign to my family, they have always respected my choice. From the first time I brought Christopher home, my mom has cooked us vegan meals and now stocks her kitchen with soymilk and other vegan staples before we visit. That is not to say it has never been difficult. The first time I came home after becoming vegan, my dad picked me up at the Sacramento airport, which is almost three hours from Redding, where my family lives. On the way home he wanted to stop for food, and sort of shrugged before saying, "I don't know what to feed you." Eventually we were able to find a place where we could both eat.

It was more difficult to explain the idea of veganism to my niece Kylie, who was about four when it came up in conversation. She and my mom were playing a computer game about dinosaurs, and my mom was explaining the difference between carnivores, omnivores, and herbivores. She explained that humans were omnivores, but as a side note added that Aunt Kerri and Uncle Christopher were herbivores. Kylie promptly asked, "Are they dinosaurs?" While there is occasional teasing—it would be impossible to grow up in my family without developing a sense of humor and a thick skin—my family has always been supportive.

Before we could dig into the desserts, my sister set aside a special tray with some cupcakes decorated to celebrate events from the past year: my grandmother's eightieth birthday, one cousin's graduation from eighth grade, my mom's and uncle Bill's retirement, another cousin's first child, and my brother-in-law's and my thirtieth birthdays. Then the cupcakes were passed around.

I had one cupcake. They were delicious as usual, but I didn't feel the need to overindulge. But by the time I finished, Christopher had already inhaled his dessert. Wiping the chocolate from his cheek, he asked, "Should I have another?"

"No," I replied. "You don't need one."

"I think I'm going to have another," he said, smiling.

"Why do you ask me if you're going to do it no matter what I say?"

"I don't know, but I'm going to have another."

I shrugged my shoulders as he navigated his way through my family members and leaned over the tray, examining which would be the best choice. Maybe he was looking for the biggest one to make a second cupcake worth it, or perhaps he wanted the one with the most frosting. Either way, it would take some time to change our habits.

Bad Brains and Barbecued Black-Eyed Peas

Christopher

I was a chubby kid during most of my childhood, and even now I struggle to maintain a healthy body weight. As a guy, this dilemma has less cultural baggage to unpack, but psychologically it can be just as haunting. I constantly debate about what to eat, how much to eat, and what to buy when we go shopping for food. However, our experiments with eating on a dollar a day and eating on the Thrifty Food Plan helped me get a better sense of the different ways I could nourish myself. As a result, I felt better prepared to enter this new era in our eating lives. Our goal to eat better and to live a more healthful lifestyle, while making choices that captured what we believe is best for the world, forced me to better understand my identity as seen through the lens of food. There are so many factors to consider when deciding what to eat that it's no wonder many of us battle with how best to feed ourselves. It's hard to know if the food we are eating is good for us, and if we really need to avoid things like saturated fats and high-fructose corn syrup. Industry-sponsored nutritionism and sound-bite journalism have only made things worse.

So this new adventure in healthy eating came with lots of new questions. If we see ourselves as people who care about the environment, can we really justify buying bell peppers grown in Holland, or shipping a cheesecake from Philadelphia? If we believe that slavery was intolerable, should we be buying chocolate? Do exploited immigrants pick our tomatoes? Is buying local really that important? Our recent experiments in eating allowed us to widen the scope of these possibilities even further, and forced me to consider how I formed my choices surrounding food in the first place. If I wanted to know why I believed what I did about mealtime, I would have to dig up my past and explore the roots of my eating life. So that is what I did.

Growing up, I spent parts of my summers working at my father's fire protection business, filing papers, shredding documents, doing inventory, and sweeping the warehouse floor. My parents were doing their best to teach me the value of a dollar, and the lesson extended after payday, when they forced me to put that money in the bank for "my future." At the time, it seemed ridiculously unfair. The fact that I spent large chunks of my summer working, and then was not allowed to spend my hard-earned dollars at the toy store, seemed patently absurd. What if I wanted to buy my own copy of the Nintendo game Mike Tyson's Punch-Out, or that cool machine that told the stories of baseball players when you put their cards in it? It was my money, and I wanted to spend it. If I had been just a few years older, I might have believed that my parents' efforts were part of some communist plot that included child labor. As an adult, I now understand their motives, and I have to admit that my work ethic and desire to save money are due in part to their tutelage. Yet the value of a dollar hit home in a more palpable way when I turned eleven years old.

During my sixth-grade year at La Costa Meadows elementary school, I was in a place familiar to many twelve-year-olds. I was about to enter middle school; I had friends, but wasn't sure what would happen when we split up to go to different schools the following year, and I was anxious about being liked by girls. This was also the year my parents divorced, and I stopped playing little league baseball. What I remember most, however, is being in Mr. Howard's class. He was the "cool" sixth-grade teacher, and I couldn't believe how lucky I was to have him. While I don't remember anything about his teaching, or the material, what I do recall is the excitement I felt when he took me and three other students to Taco Bell for lunch one day.

This was the biggest reward a student could gain in Mr. Howard's class—a special off-campus lunch trip with him on Friday afternoon. I'm not sure this practice would fly these days, but back then it was a dream come true for my classmates and me. I found out about the trip the day before, but unfortunately I forgot to mention the event to my parents (who at that point were still together). The result was that I had no money to buy my own lunch. I had never been to a Taco Bell before, but I knew that the menu items were cheap. I couldn't access my own bank account before school (not that my parents would have let me), so I scoured the house searching for loose change. I swiped a stack of quarters from my dad's dresser and pilfered my mom's purse, making sure to pick the nickels and dimes out of every nook and cranny of that oversized bag. When all was counted, I had two dollars and eighty-nine cents. I put my change in a small Ziploc bag and headed for school.

I couldn't focus that morning during class, and by the time lunch arrived, my hand was clenched tight around my small bag of coins. The car seemed to fly through our community, and I was so worried about having enough money to eat that I refrained from talking to my classmates on the way there. I remember the wind on my face and worrying about having to ask my teacher to help pay for my lunch. Finally, we pulled up to the drive-through, and while my peers ordered, I planned out every penny of my lunch budget. I settled on two beef tacos and a medium soda, and was left with just over thirty cents. This was the first time I had ever paid for my own meal, and it felt good. The fact that I could afford it, and didn't suffer an embarrassing moment in front of my cool teacher, made me proud. Although I wasn't aware of it at the time, I was beginning to shape my own food identity. This moment defined my eating habits well into my teen years.

As teenagers, my friends and I could eat a delicious meal very cheaply, and with the added benefit of newly issued drivers' licenses, hitting the drive-through became a regular part of hanging out. We were hungry growing boys, and our experiences with food were limited to family trips to the grocery store, snacking on junk food, and only having to pay for meals when we wanted to get away from the cul-de-sac. We had no idea how much more went into what we were eating. The struggles of our single mothers to provide for us—by now, many of our parents were divorced—the worker struggles involved with the tomatoes we were eating in our Taco Bell burritos, the treatment of the animals who made up the beef filling, the marketing efforts that convinced us what to eat in the first place: None of this was on our adolescent radar. We ate what we wanted, and when we wanted, without having any idea of the interconnected food web we were a part of. Information about the food system was not widely available or easy to find; not that we were looking. These were the days before wide use of the Internet, the time period that many of us refer to as B.G. (before Google).

However, as my friends and I grew up, our worldview was widened on a daily basis. The schoolteacher in me would love to say that we had great mentors who helped us see the world anew, but unfortunately this wouldn't be true. School was absolutely irrelevant, and attending classes served only one purpose: to see one another and talk about more important things. When we started going to punk shows, this became our *raison d'être*. In addition to helping us focus our angst, this community gave us access to information that we couldn't find anywhere else, information that was central to the challenges facing humanity. We might have been reading Richard Wright's *Black Boy* in English class, but this gave us little reason to focus on race issues. Following the organization Anti-Racist Action, and confronting the white supremacists at punk shows, was far more immediate.

It was through this community that we discovered the plight of animals on concentrated animal feeding operations, or "factory farms." At sixteen, this was the first time I learned where my food came from. The title of a leaflet I picked up at the Good Riddance merchandise table had a photo of a cow lying on the ground, looking up at the camera, and was titled "Downed Cow: This Story Will Change Your Life." Indeed, it did. I began thinking more about the consequences of eating meat, yet despite this, I didn't immediately change my diet.

Later on, when my friend Josh went vegetarian, I made a point of eating my meat with vigor in front of him. I thought my showy enjoyment was both original and hilarious. Yet the more reading I did, the more troubled I became by the dissonance between my love for animals like cats and dogs, and my love for eating cows, pigs, and chickens.

Over the next year or so, there were several experiences that forced me to find a solution to my internal discord. Like the time I had blood drawn after eating my value meal at McDonald's, only to see a half-inch thick white layer of fat floating at the top of the vial; or the time when I toured with a friend's band and ended up staying the night at our host's home and meeting their small pig, whose fluttering wet nose woke me up in the morning (much like my dog's). After reading more about the modern food system and the treatment of animals, reflecting on that information, and searching my core for what felt right, inevitably it was music that helped me choose to become vegetarian. Driving in the car with friends on our way to a show, I heard the song "Cats and Dogs" by Gorilla Biscuits, a quintessential hardcore band from New York. I read the lyrics in the liner notes, and the truths they described about our attitudes toward animals distilled the issue for me: We love cats and dogs, and yet we slaughter pigs, cows, and chickens, even though they also have distinct personalities and feel pain. Having recently met a pig up close, this struck a chord.

This newfound sense of clarity regarding what I ate was my first realization that what I did in the world, and how I lived, was a direct extension of what I believed. Soon after deciding to become vegetarian, I found that there were also several academic philosophical arguments supporting the rights of animals. When I gave up cheese as well, I became vegan.

Over the years, my sense of identity and my lifestyle changes eventually led to other questions about where our food comes from. I also learned that eating habits are not all that difficult to change, if you have a good enough reason to change them.

Kerri's ten-year journey to becoming a vegetarian, and then going vegan, was much different from my own. As a young woman surrounded by recreational hunters, anytime she brought up the idea of straying from a meat-centered diet, the notion was laughed off. Our different eating histories only help to underline how personal our relationships with food are. I am sure that whether you ask an ardent meat eater, a person living with celiac disease, or a devout locavore how they came to decide what is for dinner, they will each have a very individual food narrative. As stated earlier, recently we had become more keenly aware of issues like unpaid labor practices and environmental concerns related to industry.

During our experiments with low-budget menus, these issues were all starting to come into focus in a sharpened way. I knew, for instance, that eating animal products was the largest contributor to greenhouse gas emissions and global warming, but I was unaware that by choosing to be vegan, we were doing far more for both humans and the environment than even the most dedicated locavores. I knew that working in a slaughterhouse was one of the most dangerous jobs in America, where human rights abuses were rampant, but I had no idea that in Immokalee, Florida, illegally trafficked migrant workers were living in modern-day slavery. (In one documented instance, a farm worker was walking along the road and one of the labor contractors "decided the worker was probably trying to escape, forced him into their van, broke his knees with a hammer, and threw him out of the moving vehicle.") I knew that buying organic food was better for the environment, but had never considered that, as the World Health Organization reports, "Three million cases of pesticide poisoning occur every year, resulting in more than 250,000 deaths."

To learn that these issues weren't isolated but part of the larger reality involved within the modern food system was startling. No longer were we just thinking about issues like cost and convenience. Even though these remained important to us, our concerns stretched beyond our desire to lower our grocery bills; we wanted to help with hunger issues within our community.

In light of these revelations, we decided we could spend a little more on food during our healthy eating plan. Before we started the dollar diet, we bought local and organic whenever we could. But during our experiments, this ceased entirely. We were vegan, which was simple on a low-cost budget, but we still tended to overeat when we could. So the goal for the new plan was to be as healthy as possible, using our money to support practices that are best for people, animals, and the Earth itself, while not going broke. Unlike half of the world's population, we had more than $2.50 a day to live our lives, and so our challenge would be to navigate the modern global food system, to stay healthy, and to do so affordably. Through lots of reading, talking with people in our community, and transforming the way we saw our meals, we knew it was possible.

By the first week, it was clear that the largest challenge would be trying to stick to healthy eating patterns. While we learned to eat less on the dollar diet, overeating had been a continual challenge, and it was hard to give up snacks such as chips and cookies. This is one of the reasons why I decided to take a more active role in planning and preparing our meals, which prompted me to sign us up for our local CSA. I longed for a deeper connection with what we ate.

To start living this way, I needed something that would keep me interested in cooking, a task that I usually avoid. I picked up a copy of Bryant Terry's *Vegan Soul Kitchen*. My touring across the country to play music had allowed me to eat all kinds of wonderful food, but from the first time I ate soul food in the Deep South, I was crazy about it. When I planned our menu for the first few weeks of this new endeavor, I included things like Jamaican stuffed veggie pockets and barbecued black-eyed peas. Kerri had been obsessively making seared kale with a light tahini dressing, which rounded things out perfectly. I set to work cutting and chopping fresh carrots and potatoes and soaking them in a specially seasoned roux, adding peas and corn as it thickened. The warm aromas transformed the house, and Terry's recommended cooking music, a punk band known as Bad Brains, reminded me of how that community shaped my life.

I rolled out my chilled wheat flour pastry dough and scooped the filling into each pocket, pressing the edges closed with a fork. I let my black-eyed peas simmer in the homemade barbecue sauce that Kerri put together a couple days earlier, and sampled each item as I went along. As I tasted the marinated black-eyed peas, I noted that this meal was prepared with our ethics, our health, and our wallets in mind. Dried black-eyed peas are high in protein and fiber, low in fat, and at two dollars a pound, they were more than affordable—especially since we only needed a fraction of that for this meal. I wondered if this process was something we'd be able to replicate in the fall, given our busy teaching schedules.

So far, we had mostly had small fruit smoothies for breakfast, usually including frozen strawberries, bananas, and, when we had it, kale. We would use some orange juice or soymilk to give it a smooth consistency. While people in our area spend anywhere from four to six dollars for this treat, I could whip them up in minutes for a fraction of the cost. We continued to eat small servings of cereal every now and then, but we had moved on from the store-brand cornflakes in the Thrifty Food Plan and were now buying whole grain cereals that were high in fiber and protein and low in added sugars. If a cereal had a long list of ingredients we usually put it back on the shelf. When we wanted to sweeten it up, as these types of cereals can, at times, seem bland, we would add some chopped fresh strawberries or white nectarines; blueberries were also a common addition.

For lunches I tried making some new things that would be relatively easy, inexpensive, and last us for a few days. My first batch of lentil stew fit the bill perfectly. This high-protein dish was easy to put together in our Crock-Pot and, since it simmered all day, the house smelled fantastic. The crushed tomatoes and spinach gave the lentils some extra kick, and the rice helped give it a lighter texture. Since we had a good amount of lentils, we also used them in tacos, seasoning them with jalapeños, onion powder, and garlic. The recipe came from a back issue of *Home Cooking* magazine that Kerri's grandmother had sent us a year earlier. Since we were getting all kinds of produce, we often ate salads just to keep up with our CSA deliveries. When we planned to make more traditional dishes, we'd look for ways to make them healthier, like making mashed potatoes with sweet potatoes instead of russets due to their higher levels of fiber, foliates, and carotenoids (a source of vitamin A).

Kerri also prepared some inexpensive and healthy options for dinners (which ended up being lunches the next day), such as a kale soup that included barley, carrots, and garbanzo beans. All she really had to buy were those few ingredients, as she had been saving vegetable scraps in a freezer bag to make her own broth. This big batch of soup cost us about five dollars to make, and filled each of our bowls on three different occasions, coming to eighty-three cents per serving. One week, Kerri had an abundance of tomatoes and zucchinis growing in the backyard, so on Sunday night she put together dinners that would last us the whole week: vegetable lasagna; Tuscan-style pasta with chickpeas, zucchini, and rosemary; and a zucchini-chickpea-tomato curry. The lasagna, which was by far the most expensive, ended up being about $1.25 a serving, the pasta came to fifty-eight cents a serving, and the curry came in at forty-three cents a plate. Each of these dishes lasted us all week, and we ended up alternating them for lunches as well. There was so much food that Kerri took some to her friend Gail, and we sent my sister home with half of the curry leftovers.

While the cost of our healthy eating during the first few weeks had put us at about $6.80 each per day (right around the national average), this week, when we used a few ingredients for several different meals, costs went down considerably. Cereal for breakfast (including soymilk) totaled about sixty-eight cents; if we had lasagna for lunch ($1.25) and curry for dinner (forty-three cents), our daily total was about $2.36, or just under a third of the national average. Of course, this cost does not include any of Kerri's harvest. If we considered all of the garden supplies, this would have made our meals far more expensive. In addition to saving money, everything we ate was either organic, local, or both. We have posted some of our sample menus and recipes on our website for you to enjoy.

But tonight was my night to cook, and we were having Jamaican veggie pockets. Once things were ready, I scooped reasonably sized portions onto our plates. I lifted the warm pastry pocket and glanced over at Kerri. The look on her face as she took her first bite was all the validation I needed to give me confidence in this new plan. It was possible, and it would be delicious.

Overrun by Produce

....

Kerri

At the end of our first month of healthy eating, Christopher and I sat down to plan our grocery shopping for the week. It was obvious that there had been a significant change in the way we approached our weekly trips to the grocery store. Before any of our eating experiments, it wasn't uncommon for us to spend between $125 and $150 per week, or up to $600 a month for just the two of us. Often we'd fill our carts with boxes and cans of processed foods. We had now made it through the month spending $411.41, 30 percent less than before, including two weeks' worth of fresh organic produce from our CSA. We were trying new foods and working on eating healthfully. Not only that, but we were seeing that as we stocked up on staple items, we were getting fewer and fewer items at the store with each trip. Our weekly grocery bill had become progressively less expensive.

"I really liked those seitan cutlets with homemade barbecue sauce," Christopher said. I grabbed the cookbook off the shelf and flipped to find the recipe.

Scanning the ingredients, I said, "Let's see, we only need to get the chiles and some tomato sauce; we have all the other stuff."

Christopher jotted down the items. "Let's have the chard with it.

Don't you have some in your garden?" I nodded. He made a note and continued, "We have everything we need for polenta."

With the rest of the week planned, we headed out to the store with only about ten items on our list and one bag in hand. Before we started this journey, our list would have been five times as long, and we would have needed at least five or six of our canvas bags. Now things were far different.

When we walked through the door, I reflected that I felt as if half of my life had been spent wandering grocery store aisles. My decision to work at a grocery store when I was eighteen had little to do with the fact that it was my first choice, and much to do with the fact that I knew I would be hired. When I turned in my application, I was embarrassed, but my grandpa had insisted. The manager towered over me, and I was intimidated by his booming voice. I handed my application over to him with a note attached to it with a paper clip. It said: "Jim, this is my granddaughter." The manager took one look at it and let out a bellowing laugh that made me cower. "So you think this will get you a job?" He winked at me and told me he'd let me know when there was an opening.

Close to thirty years earlier, my grandfather had hired the tall teenager who worked his way up in the business and would now be my boss. Working at a grocery store seemed like a natural path for me. After five years of owning his own store, my grandfather went to work for a friend whose grocery business was expanding. He retired thirty-two years later from the corporate office of that company as one of the buyers. Because of this, my sisters and I were often the first kids in our school to have new products, as a result of samples given to my grandfather. When squeezable lunch box drinks first came out when I was in elementary school, a teacher rushed over to me because she thought I was drinking straight from a ketchup bottle. To this day, my parents still have a beach towel with a large image of a cherry-flavored Capri-Sun on it, and Campbell's soup bowls from the 1984 Winter Olympics. Perhaps this is the reason that I love soup as much as I do.

When my sisters and I were young, my dad, who is a teacher,

worked summers and holidays at a grocery store to help make ends meet. But the family connections to the grocery world do not stop there. My uncle is a manager, and my sisters have also worked in the business at one time or another. In fact, both of my sisters met their husbands while working as baggers. My mom is one of the only people on her side of the family who never worked in a grocery store, something she still holds against my grandfather, because when she wanted a job, girls were not allowed to be "box boys."

With all of this insight and experience, it seems that writing about ways to save money on food would come naturally to me, but it did not. I know that checking the markdown bins or shelves can be a quick way to save a few dollars, but through our experiments, it was continual trial and error to find out the best ways to eat a healthful and inexpensive diet. Navigating the store for the best prices and the healthiest options is something that took some time, but we now approach shopping with the confidence of professionals.

We had grabbed a basket instead of a cart to help collect our items. Now that we had reevaluated the way we approached grocery shopping, our lists were shorter and better planned out. This was in part due to what we learned during our previous experiments. While we were eating on the Thrifty Food Plan, our second shopping trip to the store that had better prices opened our eyes to the cost difference between two seemingly similar stores. While we loved our natural foods store, we were paying almost $7 for a half-gallon of soymilk, but at a chain store, we could get a gallon for only $5.99. The dollar-diet project confirmed for us that bulk foods are less expensive per ounce, and to this day we are still working our way through massive amounts of beans, flour, and cornmeal. The oatmeal, alas, is still sitting in its corner in the cupboard. Perhaps at some point I'll regain my taste for it, or at least turn it into cookies for my students.

Christopher recently used some of the oatmeal to make a batch of maple-glazed granola, and this allowed us to use something we were sick of and fashion something new. His preparation of this homemade breakfast cereal required that we pick up some maple syrup at the store, since Christopher needed more than we could reasonably pilfer from McDonald's. Pricing out maple syrup for this project was quite surprising. Our natural foods store offers about ten different versions of pure maple syrup, and the cheapest is nine dollars, for eight ounces. We simply couldn't rationalize the purchase. The chain store across the street boasted over twenty different options, but only one that was actually pure maple syrup; the rest were a blend of other sweeteners such as high-fructose corn syrup. There we were able to find an organic pure maple syrup for eight dollars, but this bottle contained twelve ounces—30 percent more than the cheapest bottle at the natural foods store. Even so, at prices like these, we'll be limiting how often we use maple syrup.

While Christopher did try making some new things like granola for breakfast, during this plan, fruit smoothies and a piece of whole grain toast with a spot of pure peanut butter became regular options.

While I may lament that we don't have a true pantry in our kitchen, in truth we have a decent-sized space for extra food. We are able to stock up on staple foods at low prices because we have the cupboard space to store them. During the dollar project, when Christopher came home with several five-gallon Home Depot buckets and informed me that they were going to sit in our kitchen, I thought he had come unhinged. They are an eyesore, and it can be frustrating to have to stack and restack buckets to find what we are looking for. However, this enabled us to buy large amounts of food at the lowest prices.

At the start of our dollar-diet project, we purchased a fifty-pound bag of flour for $15.99, whereas a typical five-pound bag might cost $2 or $3. In addition to the low price, having that raw ingredient on hand now encourages us to make things at home that we might otherwise have purchased, such as pizza dough or bread. Although it's a lot of flour to have on hand, the cost per ounce makes it a much better deal. While Christopher and I have the space to line one wall of our kitchen with buckets of flour, beans, rice, and cornmeal, it may not make sense to try it if you don't have the room; however, finding a way to make a pantry, whether in the kitchen or a closet, is essential to lowering the overall cost of eating.

I am using the term "pantry" in the sense of having a stock of staple foods that your family might consume. Pinto beans, rice, and flour are pretty common around our household, but foods that can be a base for several meals are the types of things to consider. In addition to the Home Depot buckets, we also had to rethink the way we stocked our cupboards. Instead of the boxes and cans that once filled our shelves, we now have several smaller bins with a variety of beans and grains that we use on a regular basis. There are still a few items that we buy prepackaged, like peanut butter and tofu, but we have cut back significantly, and it has made a discernible difference in how we eat and how much we spend. Now when we make our grocery lists, they often consist of fewer than ten items that we may have run out of, or a missing ingredient for a meal. In terms of healthy eating, this is helpful. I tend to be a grazer, and the way our cupboards are currently stocked, there are very few snacks, or "food-like" products, that I can just grab and munch on. This takes away the opportunity to nibble on unhealthy food all day.

As we traveled the aisles, we cruised past the end caps boasting that week's sales on chips and sodas to the canned chiles that we needed. Christopher ran to grab a carton of soymilk, as this store had the best deal, while I compared the cost of the name-brand and store-brand tomato sauce. Confirming that the store brand was the most practical, and having learned that there is little to no difference between brand names and store brands, we met at the checkout with only the items we came in for. Surprisingly, one of the simplest ways we have found to save money is to make a list and stick to it. It's easy to get lured into purchases that are unnecessary. In fact, stores count on it. The next time you're in a store, notice how many displays are offering up everything from DVDs to summer ice chests—not to mention the displays of candy and treats that are at perfect eye level for children. The worst is the checkout where people are corralled into a narrow walkway lined with tabloid magazines, candy, and even gift cards for any restaurant or store imaginable. While we waited to pay, I scanned the headlines about stars losing or gaining weight, and the latest hookups and breakups in Hollywood. Avoiding these last-minute temptations is the easiest way to help you keep costs down. Again, make a list, and buy only what you need.

Our new attitude toward the food we buy keeps costs lower, but because we are doing our cooking primarily from scratch, meal planning and preparation take extra time. While we are sticking to our commitment to eat healthfully beyond an isolated month, the challenge of balancing our time will resume again in a few weeks when the school year starts. It takes much more forethought to prepare a meal from scratch than from a box. When we start back in the fall, it will be difficult to avoid the convenience of dining out.

We have managed to cut back significantly on how frequently we go to restaurants or swing by Rico's on the way home from running errands. Currently the average American eats half of his or her meals outside the home, which is money that could be saved, or spent elsewhere. Limiting the number of meals one eats out is vital to saving money. We still dine out occasionally, but we are trying to make it more of a special occasion than a regular occurrence. Prior to our dollar-diet project, we thought little of grabbing takeout, but as expected, when we are truly looking at the cost of what we eat, it is much more expensive to eat out than to prepare food at home.

The convenience factor is a tricky one. I often feel that the benefits of eating at home aren't worth the time and effort that I have to put into preparing it. I have to remind myself that making our own meals is the healthier and less expensive option. Plus, once you have transformed your kitchen and revolutionized your habits, it's harder to go back.

When we started focusing on affordable healthy eating, we quickly learned that joining a CSA and planting a large garden meant that we would have to figure out how to use what was available at any given time.

We were filled with anticipation on the Friday when we received our first delivery of produce from our CSA, Be Wise Ranch. Our pickup point, a private residence, was only about a mile from our house, a nice walk for us and the dogs. We grabbed two bags, strapped leashes on the pups, and headed down the road. After the short walk to the house, we encountered stacks of small and large boxes filled with produce.

Since we were new to this, we had signed up for a small box on a weekly basis. But "small" is relative. We opened the box and started to place the items in our bags, cheered to discover the bounty our local farm had to offer. We were excited about everything in the box. Well, almost everything. Inside was a pound of black cherries, three cucumbers, four oranges, two grapefruit, two different kinds of lettuce, green beans, one bunch of celery, scallions, carrots, and radishes. However, lurking at the bottom of the box was a head of cabbage and five beets. To say that Christopher and I do not care for these last two items is an understatement. We had, of course, been introduced to cabbage through the Thrifty Food Plan, specifically for use in the infinitely recurring turkey-cabbage casserole and the frequent lunchtime coleslaw. Seeing the rotund green ball brought back bad memories.

The beets were another story. In the past I'd always scooped them off my salad and given them to my mom. I don't know if I had ever tried them, but the red stain that they left on my lettuce turned me off to them entirely. Christopher's first and only experience with beets still strikes a chord with him to this day. After his parents coaxed him to eat them at dinnertime, he later called his dad into the bathroom to see the blood in his poop. Christopher was panicking; standing alone in the bathroom, he feared that he would have to go to the hospital. Surprised that his son was calling him to peer at his excrement, his dad had to explain to Christopher that what he was seeing wasn't blood, but the result of the new side dish. Christopher refused to eat beets after that moment. I was glad to have an ally in my disdain for the vegetable, but this time there was no escaping them. Our thrifty sensibilities and contempt for waste would override our distaste; we would find some way to eat them.

The fact that we had all of this produce to work with helped us to change the way we planned our weekly menus. Before our adventures in eating, I usually just flipped through cookbooks trying to decide what meals I wanted to make. This gave me the chance to experiment in the kitchen in search of that enchanting new dish. While I enjoyed this process, it was time consuming, and often resulted in long lists with items that we would use only once. The one-offs would sit in the cupboard or refrigerator until Christopher would ask, "What is this for?" Things like Marsala, capers, and phyllo dough might be typical items for the resident foodie or the sophisticated urbanite, but for most people, they are far from essential.

In an effort to eat a healthier and more affordable diet, the CSA produce encouraged our new approach to shopping and eating. While the CSA posts on their website what is in a typical box each week, there are still occasional surprises, which can make it difficult to plan meals until the box arrives. This is when we started to use what now seems to be a more commonsense way of planning meals. Instead of deciding what we wanted to eat and then going shopping, we now look at what we have between our pantry and the CSA delivery to determine what we can make. So when we got our first box and found the cabbage, I was able to go online and search for recipes that I thought would make cabbage more palatable. One night we tried a stuffed cabbage recipe, and while it wasn't too bad the first night, the sizable leftovers were less appetizing.

With the beets, I made a curry sauce that I found online. The beets are roasted until they were soft enough to rub the skin off them—while it may seem obvious, I learned the hard way to give them a minute to cool down before grabbing a beet straight off the baking pan—then they are sliced and the sauce is drizzled over them. The sauce was tasty, but not enough to disguise the fact that I was still eating the dreaded beets.

By the third week of our CSA, we were beginning to be overrun with produce. Christopher was out of town, and there was no way that just one person could eat it all. I threw together a pasta dish that I named "Whatever Came in the CSA Box Pasta." It included eggplant, green beans, leeks, onion, celery, and peas (which did not come in our CSA, but which, for some reason, we had three unopened bags of in our freezer). I ate it with a side salad that used up as much lettuce as I could, as well as any vegetables that wouldn't work in the pasta dish. More beets had arrived that week, but I offloaded them on Christopher's mom, who was thrilled to get them.

When Christopher came back, one of the first things I said after hello was "We need to change our pickups to every other week." There was no point in getting more produce than we could use. It didn't matter if it was priced well if the food went to waste. Going through our refrigerator's produce drawer and pulling out almost-liquid cucumbers or blackening lettuce juxtaposed in my mind with that past September when we would have done anything for fresh produce. This furthered my desire to use all of the vegetables that crossed our threshold. It took a few weeks to figure out just how much produce would be coming, and how much we could eat. We changed our order to a large box every other week, which was a much more manageable amount.

Without a strict food budget, Christopher and I felt less isolated. We had the freedom to join friends who invited us out, and to invite them to our home. However, we still paid attention to the cost of our food and what we were eating. When I sent out an invitation to my friends for a "Stitch and Bitch" party, I was faced with the challenge of preparing snacks and appetizers for friends while keeping the cost down and the menu healthy. My girlfriends were invited to bring crocheting and knitting projects over (the stitching) while we snacked and chitchatted (the bitching). I knew that I wanted to serve appetizers, but I wanted to avoid the chips and dips that are typical party fare. This brought up all of my old urges to prepare memorable food for guests.

Rummaging through the kitchen and the garden, I did a quick survey of what was available. As I mentioned earlier, I had had no concept of how much to plant, and at this point, the first of my seventeen tomato plants was starting to produce. I picked four or five ripe ones off the vine and moved on to the basil. Following my mom's advice, I pinched back the flowers to extend the life of the plant and then clipped off a handful of leaves. The pot next to the basil contained bright green mint sprigs. The mint had taken a while to get started; I had planted it the year before in my first attempt at gardening, and it had just taken off a few months earlier. I cut a few stems. Out front where the fig tree and a lemon tree have existed for years, I picked as many lemons as I could reach and then went crawling around under the fig tree, emerging with ten cradled in my shirt. Bringing the bounty inside, I placed it on the kitchen counter. I separated the produce into piles and started planning the menu. I had ideas for most of the items, but I didn't know what to do with figs, so I started researching some recipes.

On the day of my get-together, I set out bruschetta with fresh basil and tomatoes, baked figs glazed with balsamic vinegar, and a cucumber salad with mint and lime. As my guests arrived, I showed them where to drop their crochet bags and ushered them in. My friends dove into the food with exclamations of delight. Anytime a group of teachers get together, the conversation quickly turns to talk of the school year: rumors about the upcoming year, hysterical or horrifying moments from our classrooms. While some crocheting did take place, we spent the evening conversing. Every once in a while, someone would get up to grab another piece of bruschetta or more salad. It was a hot day, and we cooled off with a sparkling rosemary lemonade. With the help of the garden and our pantry, I served my eight guests for under thirty dollars. It was inexpensive, healthy, and satisfying—everything we had been searching for.

Epilogue: Finding Our Way

Christopher

Every summer, Kerri and I have the opportunity to spend a week with her family at Donner Lake, a small area near Sierra Nevada, just northwest of Lake Tahoe. This area is perhaps most famous for the group of thirty-three led by George Donner in nine covered wagons, who in the winter of 1846 got stuck in the snow on their way to California. After a while, a group of fifteen fashioned some snow-shoes and did their best to seek help, but the blizzard got worse, and after a few people died, the remaining members of the team resorted to cannibalism in order to stay alive. Our journey to Donner Lake was nowhere near as dramatic, but it was on our most recent trip that I started to finally make sense of everything that Kerri and I had done over the past year during our eating adventures.

One afternoon on a hike in the mountains with Kerri's father, Mike, he asked, "What do you guys think about those sports drinks?" I told him that I thought they were probably fine, and that what mattered more than the individual foods or beverages were entire eating patterns. I told him that those drinks were really nothing more than sugar-water with some salt, but as long as he wasn't drinking them all the time, I thought he'd be all right. This seemed to make sense to him.

While we continued making our way through the woods, Mike went on to tell us about his experiences as a runner, and how sports drinks could be helpful. He told us about how some of his former coaches required him to eat salt tablets while training for a meet. It made me recall all of the recommendations that I had heard from some of my own coaches growing up: "Load up on pasta tonight, so you'll have energy for the game tomorrow," and teachers reminding me to "Eat a good breakfast, so you will be ready for the test." We started sharing stories about how people eat. We talked about those who can eat fast food on a regular basis and seem to maintain good health. We talked about the genetics that determine things like obesity and differing metabolisms. We talked about how for some people, avoiding fat and sugar-laden desserts was no problem, but for me, it was a serious struggle.

Pushing up a small hill, the conversation carried on into school lunch programs, and how schools make junk food available to students on a regular basis, through vending machines and foods like pizza and chicken nuggets. We talked about how even in California, where many districts have eliminated sodas, they have replaced them with equivalents that contain just as much added sugar. Kerri related a story about a friend of ours who was told by the school not to pack junk foods in her daughter's lunch anymore, only to be surprised later on by all manner of sweets and sodas at a fellow student's in-class birthday celebration.

This led us to consider the psychological baggage that comes with deciding what to eat. Birthday parties have the effect of making an emotional link between having fun and eating high-calorie foods like cake and pizza. As we talked, it became clear how interrelated and messy the food conversation really is. We joined the food dialogue because we started to feel anxious at the checkout counter, as each beep of the grocery store scanner took more from our wallets. Initially, we just wanted to save some money.

Throughout this book, we have written about our experiences while trying to eat for less: first by attempting to survive on a dollar a day; next by exploring issues of hunger and health through the

Thrifty Food Plan and food stamps; and finally by planning healthy, affordable, and ethical menus. We learned that in order to get the most for your money, you must have a lot of other things going for you as well. Income, transportation, time, education, health, location, and other factors play a role in determining what someone is able to eat. We did the best we could, given our situations; at this point, our quest is nowhere near its conclusion. However, we have come to understand that what makes the most sense for us is to sit down and plan out a menu each week. So that is what we strive to do. We base our menu on what is in our pantry, what we have from our CSA, what is in our garden, what our schedules look like for the week, and how we are feeling. This has kept us from always having snack foods in reach, and from dining out too frequently; it also allows us to reflect on a consistent basis about how we are eating.

This method has enabled us not only to save money but to evaluate our personal health, and to slowly unravel how we are connected to the food system. It has also helped us come to terms with how gender roles play out in our relationship, and how we treat each other. There were times when the sound of slammed cupboard doors spoke for us, and some silly instances that we will not soon forget, like the time Kerri stripped down to her underwear so that she wouldn't have to run back out to the store to pick up pasta. Now when she asks me to go back out for something, I can no longer make the excuse "I'm in my underwear!"

More than anything, these experiments have been incredibly humbling experiences, and they will stay with us for the rest of our lives. We used to go through each day eating when we pleased, giving little thought to the food that crossed our lips. But when you are counting every pinto bean, and picking each grain of rice from your plate after a long day at work, it has a leveling effect. Eating is no longer something that you take for granted. When you are struggling to decide how to ration your food so that it will last you through the end of the month, any concerns over personal health become echoes in the distance. Hunger takes over, and things like peanut butter seem decadent.

Over the last year, we have been hyperaware of how our privilege has allowed us to do this type of experimentation, and we have consistently tried to understand why there are *thirty-six million people* in our country who do not have much choice when it comes to deciding what and when to eat—all of them limited by the amount of money they have, and the food that is available to them. We have met with dedicated hunger activists, visited low-income neighborhoods, and restricted our own spending, in hopes of gaining some insight into the struggles that people in our nation and across the globe face on a daily basis. We've tried to stop assuming that we understand the hardships that face those who are going without. Our own families and some of our dearest friends have shared with us their struggles to eat on food stamps, and yet we can only begin to plumb the depths of these issues. Right now, as you are reading this, there are thirteen million children suffering from hunger, malnutrition, and food insecurity in the United States. We want to know why. We have tried to understand why there are a billion people worldwide who actually live on a dollar a day. We continue to try to bridge the disconnect between the fact that half of all children will be born into poverty, and the rise of childhood obesity in America.

While Mike, Kerri, and I hiked the forest, we wandered down a different trail and got lost. It took us a few minutes to find our way back, and since Kerri's dad forgot his GPS watch, we had to do things the old-fashioned way and trace our footprints. Being in the woods and not knowing exactly how to find our way out was a little frightening at first, but once we calmed down, we realized it only took common sense to track our way back to our original path.

I wondered if we could do something similar with the way we feed ourselves. Somewhere along the line, possibly during the agricultural revolution, ten thousand years ago, our culture strayed from how it used to eat, and some important wisdom was lost along the way. We all need to explore the roots of how we eat, in order to find our way back to good health.

Our choice to eat whole grains and fresh fruits and vegetables, instead of foodlike products such as frozen burritos and prepackaged snacks, comes from understanding that we are the sole protectors of our bodies, and from the recognition that food companies do not have our best interests at heart. It has been hard letting go of cookies and crackers, but our choice to eat less, and to eat only what we need, is our way of resisting the push to overeat, and to avoid obesity. Kerri has learned that we are not professional wrestlers, and the amount on our plates doesn't need to match theirs. I've learned to live without eating sweets every single day. Joining our local CSA is one way that we can support farmers, workers, and our local economy. We decided that buying a bell pepper from Holland makes about as much sense as flying there to poop it out.

The food justice movement is growing. There are all kinds of people involved in an infinite number of ways: from city planners to organizers of school-led food drives; from mom bloggers to grassroots activists; from groups like Food Not Bombs to federal food program officials. The diversity of this movement is one of its greatest strengths. If you're reading this book, you're probably interested in such issues. We are just asking you to become consciously involved.

If you're a gardener, consider planting a row purely for donation to your local food bank (Kerri is working on this right now). If you're a teacher, help your students understand where their food comes from. If you're a doctor, help your patients understand that what and how much they eat will greatly impact their health. If you work in law enforcement, track down those who are exploiting immigrant laborers. If you are an elected official, do not be afraid to risk your reputation; if you do what is right, your constituents will eventually come around.

For everyone else: Do something. If we are each doing all that we can, solutions will start to appear. They may work only for your community, like the work of our Community Resource Center, or for thousands of people in Bangladesh, like the work of Muhammad Yunus. You won't know until you start, so break out of your routine. Life is too short to worry about how much stuff you can own, or how powerful you can become. The most memorable figures in history are those who were just regular people who decided to try something different, to turn their own lives into experiments for good. Anyone can do that; it doesn't have to cost a thing. Gandhi once said, "Almost everything you do will seem insignificant, but it is important that you do it." This applies now more than ever. Only you know what you can do—and by all means, make sure it is something you enjoy, that it is rewarding, and that it is making this world a better place.

Finding our way back down the hill from our hike, I looked at the smile on Kerri's face. We had made it out alive, before nightfall when the bears come out to, well, eat. When we got lost, we could have yelled at one another about whose fault it was, or argued about the best way to move forward, but we didn't. We looked around and searched for a solution. This is what we all must do right now. In order to meet the world's most pressing challenges, we will need to harness the best of human qualities. So please, use your own joy, your laughter, your honesty, your determination, your compassion, your ingenuity, your curiosity, and every fiber of your being. It will take nothing less.

A Dozen Ways to Save

Plan a menu. If you plan your menu for one to two weeks at a time, you will make fewer trips to the store and spend less money each time. In addition, planning meals that use similar ingredients may cut down on waste. For example, if you are making stir-fry one night, plan to toss any leftover veggies into a salad as a side dish with another meal, or use them to liven up a plain pasta dish.

Make a list and stick to it. Don't wander around the store. The longer you're there, the more money you will spend. Grocery stores are designed to make you have to walk through aisles of products to get to common household items such as milk. Stick to your mission. This will help you cut down on impulse buys and lower your grocery bill. There is a reason why high-ticket items are on display near the register.

Start a pantry. By this, we mean stock up on staple foods that are frequently used in your household and can be a base for a variety of meals. This way you can buy extra when you find a good price.

Buy in bulk. Always check the cost per ounce if your supermarket provides that information on the tags, or take a calculator with you so that you can figure out the best deal. Usually (but not always), larger sizes have better prices per ounce or unit. However, don't get tricked into buying large items just because they are inexpensive: If it isn't something you will use all of, don't buy it.

Share. If it is not affordable to buy large sizes, or you don't have the storage space for twenty-five-pound bags, go in with a friend or two and split the cost and the product.

Compare prices of name brands to store and third-party (generic) brands. Name brands are often many times more expensive, and the taste and quality of the generic brands are, in most cases, nearly identical to their more costly counterparts. In addition, check out the day-old or markdown shelves.

Only buy the produce that you can use in a week or two. If you buy produce for the whole month, it may spoil before you get to it. It doesn't matter if it was inexpensive if it was thrown out.

Waste nothing. Consider using odds and ends that might be thrown out to replace premade items like broth for soups. For instance, the broth we used to buy was almost three dollars for one quart. We started using bouillon cubes, which were much less expensive, but high in sodium. By saving veggie peels, ends, and stalks, you can create your own broth. We toss all of ours into a Ziploc bag and freeze it until we are ready to cook. There are recipes online, or you can skim the recipes and then just experiment with what you have saved.

Eat in season. In-season produce can be less expensive. If you are adventurous and willing to experiment with in-season veggies that you may not have tried before, find out if there is a CSA (community-supported agriculture) farm in your area that you can join.

Don't get stuck shopping at only one store. Compare prices at different stores to find the one that consistently has the lower prices on the items you buy most often. If a store is having a great sale on an item you use frequently, check it out, but only purchase what you go in for. Sales are designed to lure you into the store so that you will buy more than just that product. If you buy impulse items, it may defeat the purpose of your trip.

Eat at home most of the time. Eating out is far more expensive and far less healthy than preparing food at home.

Choose one day a week to do the bulk of your cooking. If you take the time to cook several meals in one day, you can freeze or refrigerate items to be eaten over the course of a week or two. Having prepared meals at home may help to cut down on the temptation to eat out after a long day at work.

Sowing the Seeds of Progress

There are many ways that you can get involved to help others. Whether you're looking to donate money or become a full-fledged activist, there are plenty of opportunities for you to consider. We recommend that you ask yourself what you're most passionate about, and what you enjoy doing, and then find a way to merge those interests with your activism. While making your plans, here are some suggestions.

Stay informed. Make reading about these issues part of your routine. If you use a homepage that aggregates blogs and news information, add feeds that are specifically geared toward these issues. Subscribing to e-mail lists and publications from the organizations that work on these concerns will make staying on top of developments effortless.

Know your community. Take some time to understand what issues are facing your area. Then search for organizations that are involved in these issues and see what they are up to. Ask your family, friends, and colleagues if they are familiar with any groups already working on projects that you are interested in. If no groups exist in your town or city, search for statewide groups, and then national organizations.

Be the message. There is a much-quoted anecdote about Gandhi, in which a reporter was following him as he was being taken off to prison. The reporter asked, "Gandhi, what is your message?" His alleged reply was, "My life is my message." As you do this work, be aware that how you live is more important than what you say.

Take action. No matter what you can do, do something. It may feel small and insignificant, but it is important that you do it. Consider your actions as moving the rudder on a ship. Over time, even a small turn to the right will have dramatic consequences. You could end up somewhere that you never expected.

Have fun. Regardless of what you decide to do, if you're not enjoying it, then it is very likely that you will burn out, turn off others, and resent the issue you are working on. There are plenty of people in the world who are no fun to be around; don't be one of them. While things may get tough, be reflective and keep a positive attitude.

IN THE SHORT TERM

If you're looking for things you can do right away, consider transforming your kitchen by stocking it with healthy foods (if there are health claims on the packaging, they might not be that healthy); writing your elected representatives and asking them to get involved with hunger and food justice issues; donating your time to a local organization; donating 1 to 5 percent of your income to a group fighting extreme poverty; planting a garden (and establishing a row just to share with your local food bank); shopping with your principles guiding you (go vegan, buy fair trade, buy local, buy organic, etc.); using sites like Facebook to post stats and stories related to these issues; or thinking of your own experiment that you can conduct and share with others.

Here are just a few of the organizations we think deserve your attention:

Community Food Security Coalition
3830 SE Division Street
Portland, OR 97202
(503) 954-2970
www.foodsecurity.org

The Community Food Security Coalition (CFSC) is a North American coalition of diverse people and organizations working from the local to international levels to build community food security. Their membership includes almost three hundred organizations from social and economic justice, anti-hunger, environmental, community development, sustainable agriculture, community gardening, and other fields. They are dedicated to building strong, sustainable local and regional food systems that ensure access to affordable, nutritious, and culturally appropriate food to all people at all times. They seek to develop self-reliance among all communities in obtaining their food and to create a system of growing, manufacturing, processing, making available, and selling food that is regionally based and grounded in the principles of justice, democracy, and sustainability.

Food Research and Action Center
875 Connecticut Avenue, NW, Suite 540
Washington, DC 20009
(202) 986-2200
www.frac.org

The Food Research and Action Center (FRAC) is the leading national nonprofit organization working to improve public policies and public-private partnerships to eradicate hunger and undernutrition in the United States. FRAC works with hundreds of national, state, and local nonprofit organizations, public agencies, and corporations to address hunger and its root cause, poverty.

Institute for Food and Development Policy

398 60th Street

Oakland, CA 94618

(510) 654-4400

www.foodfirst.org

The purpose of the Institute for Food and Development Policy is to eliminate the injustices that cause hunger. Called one of the country's "most established food think tanks" by *The New York Times*, the Institute for Food and Development Policy, also known as Food First, is a "people's" think tank. They carry out research, analysis, advocacy, and education for informed citizen engagement with the institutions and policies that control production, distribution, and access to food. Their work both informs and amplifies the voices of social movements fighting for food sovereignty: people's right to healthy and culturally appropriate food produced through ecologically sound and sustainable methods, and their right to define their own food and agriculture systems—at home and abroad.

Oxfam America

226 Causeway Street, 5th Floor

Boston, MA 02114-2206

www.oxfamamerica.org

Oxfam America is an international relief and development organization that creates lasting solutions to poverty, hunger, and injustice. Together with individuals and local groups in more than one hundred countries, Oxfam saves lives, helps people overcome poverty, and fights for social justice. They are an affiliate of Oxfam International. Their vision is a just world without poverty.

World Hunger Year (WHY)
505 Eighth Avenue, Suite 2100
New York, NY 10018
1-800-5-HUNGRY
www.whyhunger.org

Founded in 1975, WHY is a leader in the fight against hunger and poverty in the United States and around the world. WHY is convinced that solutions to hunger and poverty can be found at the grassroots level. WHY advances long-term solutions to hunger and poverty by supporting community-based organizations that empower individuals and build self-reliance, i.e., offering job training, education, and after-school programs; increasing access to housing and health care; providing microcredit and entrepreneurial opportunities; teaching people to grow their own food; and assisting small farmers. WHY connects these organizations to funders, media, and legislators.

Acknowledgments

This book would not be around if it weren't for the hard work of several people and organizations. Before we thank those who played more specific roles in bringing this text to the world, we would especially like to thank the Community Resource Center in Encinitas, Food Not Bombs, the San Diego Farm Bureau, the San Diego Caring Council, the Supportive Parents Information Network (SPIN), and the International Rescue Committee (San Diego), for all they do to help people amidst a shameful excuse for a "safety net," and who helped us understand the dynamics of poverty, hunger, food insecurity, and the SNAP program. We are especially grateful to Jennifer Tracy of the San Diego Hunger Coalition for taking the time to sit down with us until all of our questions were answered. We also want to thank the groups who supported the "Cultivating Food Justice" conference in San Diego during May 2009, and the individuals who organized it. The work of these groups in our community, and of those like them, is both humbling and inspiring.

We'd like to thank the readers of our blog who shared their stories with us, challenged our thinking, and were willing to help us raise money for the Community Resource Center in the fall of 2008; because of you, someone was able to get a little something to eat. Without the article written by Tara Parker-Pope at *The New York Times*, the rest of the world might not ever have heard of what we were doing, and to all the journalists whose work followed hers, we are thankful that you took the time to ask thoughtful, engaging questions, and usually wrote thoughtful, honest pieces about our project.

Without our literary agent, Lynn Johnston, we probably wouldn't have written this book in the first place, and her work in helping us find a suitable home for its release has been essential to everything we have wanted to do. Without the help of our colleagues Suzi VanSteenbergen, Erika Wanczuck, and David Andrew Tow, our editor would have had far more work to do. Thanks to them for reading various drafts and chapters of this book; their thoughtful comments helped us fix this thing as we went along. To our editor, Leslie Wells at Hyperion, thanks for guiding us through our first book, challenging us to do better, and making this text what it is today. We'd like to thank our publicist, Allison McGeehon, as well as all the folks at Hyperion who believed in our book and have worked like crazy to get it out so quickly.

We owe a great debt to all of the writers and scholars whose work helped us along the way: Joel Berg, John Bowe, Faith D'aluisio, Barbarah Ehrenreich, Barry Glassner, Sandor Ellix Katz, Bill and Ruth Kaysing, David A. Kessler, Harvey Levenstein, Peter Menzel, Marion Nestle, Raj Patel, Michael Pollan, Leon Rappoport, Paul Roberts, Eric Schlosser, Loretta Schwartz-Nobel, Bryant Terry, Mark Winne, and many more who took on the task of writing about food, economics, poverty, health, nutrition, psychology, and every other discipline that seeks to unravel the complexities of what is (or isn't) for dinner.

We'd like to thank Sylvia at Sipz Cafe and the staff at Rico's taco shop for feeding us when we were too tired to cook.

Christopher would like to thank all of the punk and hardcore kids, free thinkers, artists, and teachers whose visionary work continues to influence this book and all else that he does. In particular the work of REFUSED, Fugazi, At the Drive-In, Good Riddance,

Rise Against, By the Grace of God, Boysetsfire, Philip Glass, Ani Difranco, Saul Williams, Jackson Pollock, Andy Warhol, Gregory Colbert, Noam Chomsky, Daniel Quinn, M. K. Gandhi, William DeJean, Gail Zides, Saturday James, Zoe Weil and the Institute for Humane Education, Dr. Tara Sethia and the Ahimsa Center, Steve Elliott and the Walter Cronkite School of Journalism and Mass Communication at Arizona State University, Peta2.com, The Che Cafe, 924 Gilman Street, Robert Pennington, Patrick Conway, Pulin Modi, Spencer Gooch, and Eric Davis. XXX.

Kerri would like to thank Mary Nobel, who pushed her to take her first great adventure in life; Brian McCall, for being an inspiring teacher; and Nicole Love, for the daily phone calls and continued strength.

Of course, no list of acknowledgments would be complete without recognizing our families for all of their love and support, our friends for keeping us grounded, and our students for giving us a reason to wake up in the morning (most of the time). And to Viola, Horatio, and Mrs. B., even though you'll never be able to read this, your unrelenting love for us made writing this book that much easier.

Notes

CHAPTER 2

Page 20

U.S. food supply increased: Nestle, Marion. *Food Politics: How the Food Industry Influences Health and Nutrition.* University of California Press. Berkeley. 2002.

high-calorie, energy-dense foods: Drewnowski and Monsivais. "The Rising Cost of Low-Energy-Density Foods." *Journal of the American Dietetic Association.* Volume 107, Number 12. December 2007.

Page 24

"supermarket redlining": Patel, Raj. *Stuffed & Starved: The Hidden Battle for the World Food System.* Melville House Publishing. Brooklyn, NY. 2008.

CHAPTER 3

Page 33

Food Not Bombs: "The Story of Food Not Bombs." Accessed September 2, 2009. http://www.foodnotbombs.net/story.html

Page 34

grocery store auctions: Rubinkam, Michael. "Thrifty shoppers 'Sold!' on grocery auctions: Bidders are willing to take some food that is past its sell-by date." March 25, 2009. MSNBC.com. Accessed June 5, 2009. http://www.msnbc.msn.com/id/29865090/

CHAPTER 4
Page 45
including Campbell's Soup: U.S. News & World Report. February 15, 1957.

the "gift of time": Alexander McFarlane. "Of Convenience, Food Innovation, and Calling the Tune: The Revolutionary Imperative." *Food Technology.* Issue 23 (April 1969).

Page 46
two and a half hours: Patel, Raj. *Stuffed & Starved: The Hidden Battle for the World Food System.* Melville House Publishing. Brooklyn, NY. 2008.

CHAPTER 5
Page 55
enriched foods: Nestle, Marion. *Food Politics: How the Food Industry Influences Health and Nutrition.* University of California Press. Berkeley. 2002.

idea of enriching foods: Wilson, M. L. "Nutrition and Defense," *Journal of the American Dietetic Association* 17 (January 1947): 13–14.

CHAPTER 6
Page 72
thirty-six million people: Berg, Joel. *All You Can Eat: How Hungry Is America?* Seven Stories Press. New York. 2008.

CHAPTER 7
Page 80
Greater Philadelphia's Coalition Against Hunger: Greater Philadelphia Coalition Against Hunger. "News and Media Coverage." 2006. Accessed March 15, 2006. http://www.hungercoalition.org/hungerinfo/ newsandmedia/index.html

Oregon governor Theodore R. Kulongoski: Yardly, William. "A Governor Truly Tightens His Belt." *The New York Times.* May 1, 2007. Accessed March 20, 2009. http://www.nytimes.com/2007/05/01/us/01stamps .html

several members of Congress: Congressional Food Stamp Challenge. "U.S. Members of Congress Live on a Food Stamp Budget." October 30, 2007. Accessed March 15, 2009. http://foodstampchallenge.typepad.com/

Page 81
Supplemental Nutrition Assistance Program (SNAP): Denice, Karen. "Eating Healthy on a Shoestring Budget." CNN. March 6, 2009. Accessed March 20, 2009. http://www.cnn.com/2009/HEALTH/03/06/callebs .eating.food.stamps/index.html

The Economic Research Service: Clauson, Annette. "Despite Higher Food Prices, Percent of U.S. Income Spent on Food Remains Constant." *AmberWaves.* September 2008. Accessed July 3, 2009. http://www.ers. usda.gov/AmberWaves/september08/findings/percentofincome/htm

average low-income . . . household Economic Research Service. Food CPI and Expenditures: Table 7. USDA. June 17, 2008. Accessed June 3, 2009. http://www.ers.usda.gov/briefing/CPIFoodandExpenditures/Data/table7.htm2009

Page 82

national average food stamp benefit Center for Nutrition Policy and Promotion. "Recipes and Tips for Healthy, Thrifty Meals." USDA. 2000. Accessed February 15, 2009. http://www.cnpp.usda.gov/Publications/FoodPlans/MiscPubs/FoodPlansRecipeBook.pdf

USDA Thrifty Food Plan Guthrie, Joanne F., Elizabeth Frazao, Margaret Andrews, and David Smallwood. "Improving Food Choices—Can Food Stamps Do More?" *AmberWaves.* Economic Research Service. April 2007. 5.2. http://www.ers.usda.gov/AmberWaves/April07/Features/Improving.htm

sample menus, forty recipes USDA. "Supplemental Nutrition Assistance Program: Fact Sheet on Resources, Income and Benefits." USDA Food and Nutrition Service. July 8, 2009. Accessed August 3, 2009. http://www.fns.usda.gov/fsp/applicant_recipients/fs_Res_Ben_Elig.htm

CHAPTER 9

Page 105

Tracy, Jennifer. San Diego Hunger Coalition. Interview. July 24, 2009.

food stamp participation "Eligibility and Issuance Requirements." California's department of social services FAQ. http://www.dss.cahwnet.gov/foodstamps/PG846.htm

Page 106

state's participation SPIN. "Barriers to Food Stamps." San Diego. Lecture. August 26, 2009.

Page 107

support the community: Bolduan, Kate, and Lesa Jansen. "Food Stamps Offer Best Stimulus." CNNMoney. January 29, 2008. Accessed July 7, 2009. http://money.cnn.com/2008/01/29/news/economy/stimulus_analysis/index.htm

farmers market: "Building the Community." City Heights Farmers
   Market. 2009. Accessed July 8, 2009. http://cityheightsfarmersmarket
   .com/wb/pages/building-the-community.php

CHAPTER 10
Page 112
"The Women in Your Lives": Husted, Marjorie. "The Women in Your Lives."
   Transcript of speech. October 13, 1952. Husted Papers, Folder 2.

Page 114
"Stamp Out Hunger" day: Levenstein, Harvey. *Paradox of Plenty: A Social
   History of Eating in Modern America.* University of California Press.
   Berkeley, Los Angeles, and London. 2003.

Page 115
the work of Joel Berg: Berg, Joel. *All You Can Eat: How Hungry Is America?*
   Seven Stories Press. New York. 2008.

Page 116
Winne's analysis: Winne, Mark. *Closing the Food Gap: Resetting the Table in
   the Land of Plenty.* Beacon Press. Boston. 2008.

Page 117
article by Mike Hughlett: Hughlett, Mike. "Grocery Inflation Likely to
   Ease in 2009." *Chicago Tribune.* December 26, 2008. Accessed July 6,
   2009. http://archives.chicagotribune.com/2008/dec/26/business/chi-fri-
   outlook-food-dec26

Page 118
shrunk the size of the jar: Martin, Andrew. "Ate a Whole Pint? Check
   Again." *The New York Times.* September 13, 2008. Accessed July 6,
   2009. http://www.nytimes.com/2008/09/14/business/14feed.html?_r=1&
   partner=permalink&exprod=permalink
"Poor? Pay Up.": Brown, DeNeen. "Poor? Pay Up." *The Washington Post.*
   May 18, 2009. Accessed July 6, 2009. http://www.washingtonpost.com/
   wp-dyn/content/article/2009/05/17/AR2009051702053.html

CHAPTER 12
Page 130
USDA needs to reconsider: "Food Stamp Recipients: A Profile." Food
   Research and Action Center. Accessed July 7, 2009. http://www.frac.org/
   html/federal_food_programs/programs/fsp_faq.html#2

Page 132
average family on food stamps: "Official USDA Food Plans: Cost of Food at Home at Four Levels, U.S. Average, April 2009." USDA Center for Nutrition Policy and Promotion. April 2009. http://www.cnpp.usda .gov/usdafoodcost-home.htm

Page 135
our area is far different: "Fast Facts: Encinitas." San Diego Association of Governments (San Diego's Regional Planning Agency). 2007. Accessed July 8, 2009. http://www.sandag.org/resources/demographics_and_other_ data/demographics/fastfacts/enci.htm

Page 136
City Heights: "Community Health Atlas for Mid-City San Diego." San Diego Health and Human Services Agency. March 2004.
both areas of San Diego: "Building the Community." City Heights Farmers Market. 2009. Accessed July 8, 2009. http://cityheightsfarmersmarket .com/wb/pages/building-the-community.php

CHAPTER 13
Page 152
Michelle Obama started a garden: Burros, Marian. "Obamas Prepare to Plant White House Vegetable Garden." *The New York Times.* March 19, 2009. http://www.nytimes.com/2009/03/20/dining/20garden.html

CHAPTER 14
Page 163
"Downed Cow": "Downed Cow: This Story Will Change Your Life." People for the Ethical Treatment of Animals. Accessed September 2, 2009. http://www.goveg.com/downedcow.asp

Page 164
global warming: "Livestock's Long Shadow: Environmental Issues and Options." United Nations, Food and Agriculture Organization, Rome. 2006. http://www.fao.org/docrep/010/a0701e/a0701e00.htm
working in a slaughterhouse: Roberts, Paul. "Spoiled: Our Industrial Food System." *Mother Jones.* April 2009.
Immokalee, Florida: "Blood, Sweat, and Fear: Workers' Rights in U.S. Meat and Poultry Plants." Investigative report. New York. Human Rights Watch. 2005. http://www.hrw.org/en/reports/2005/01/24/blood-sweat-and-fear

modern-day slavery: Bowe, John. *Nobodies: Modern American Slave Labor and the Dark Side of the New Global Economy.* Random House. New York. 2007.

Page 165
$2.50 a day: Ross, Jen. "Paying the Price for Growth." *Toronto Star.* January 8, 2005, F5. Quoted from "The Revolution Will Not Be Microwaved: Inside America's Underground Food Movements" by Sandor Ellix Katz. Chelsea Green Publishing Company. Vermont. 2006.
36 million people: Shah, Anup. "Poverty Facts & Stats." Accessed September 2, 2009. http://www.globalissues.org/article/26/poverty-facts-and-stats

CHAPTER 16
Page 181
thirteen million children: Berg, Joel. *All You Can Eat: How Hungry Is America?* Seven Stories Press. New York. 2008.
a billion people worldwide: Cauthen, Nancy, and Sarah Fass. "Who Are America's Poor Children?" National Center for Children in Poverty. November 2007. Accessed September 2, 2009. http://www.nccp.org/publications/pub_787.html

Index

About the Authors

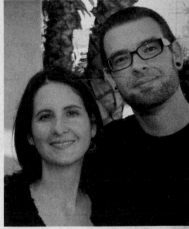

Photo © David Andrew Tow

Christopher Greenslate teaches English, social justice, and journalism to high school students in San Diego. He founded the social justice program in the school district as a forum for students to act on important issues of the day. The dollar-a-day project grew out of his desire to show his students how to get people to see an issue with a new perspective. He was a 2008 Reynolds Institute Fellow of the American Society of Newspaper Editors. He has led workshops at large events such as the annual Teachers for Social Justice Conference and the National High School Journalism Convention. Christopher was selected by Rotary International to travel to East Africa as part of a group exchange in 2009.

Kerri Leonard grew up in northern California in a family of grocers and worked at a grocery store for six and a half years. Kerri teaches English and speech and debate in San Diego County. She was named Speech and Debate Coach of the Year in San Diego.

Christopher and Kerri live in Encinitas, California.